DR. BRUCE LOWELL'S
FAT PERCENTAGE
FINDER

The New, Easy-to-Use System for Measuring the Fat in Your Diet

Bruce K. Lowell, M.D.

A Perigee Book

This book is dedicated to Diane, Jennifer,
Matt, and to the memory of my father,
Murray Lowell, who taught me to
jump the hurdles of life.

Perigee Books
are published by
The Putnam Publishing Group
200 Madison Avenue
New York, NY 10016

Library of Congress Cataloging-in-Publication Data
Lowell, Bruce K., date.
[Fat finder]
Dr. Bruce Lowell's fat percentage finder: the new, easy-to-use
system for measuring the fat in your diet/by Bruce K. Lowell.
p. cm.
ISBN 0-399-51653-0
1. Food—Fat content—Tables. I. Title.
TX553.L5L68   1991   90-39530 CIP
641.1'4—dc20

Cover design © 1991 by Bob Silverman

Printed in the United States of America
6 7 8 9 10

ACKNOWLEDGMENTS

Dr. Bruce Lowell's Fat Percentage Finder has only one author, but it would not have been possible without the work and support of my family, the members of the "team" at Weight Risk Management and Putnam books.

First, there's the love and support of my family. Diane, my wife, has been a contributor, source of insight, and the guiding force in this project. Jennifer, my daughter, gave up her Saturdays to research new foods in the local supermarkets. Matthew, my five-year-old, gave up his time with dad so this work could be completed. He continuously asked, "When is this book going to be done anyway?"

Thanks to Gracie, my office manager, who put up with my craziness. The educational staff, Lancene Union and Jill Malden, R.D., C.S.W., who helped with the food lists and always offered their comments, both good and bad.

A special thanks for the cooperation of the food manufacturers and restaurants whose information is found within this book.

Judy Linden, my editor at Putnam, whose insight and help has brought this book to fruition. I thank her for her patience and help. Jody Beard whose help was much appreciated in editing Part One. Lastly, thanks to my agents, Marrisa Smith and Eric Kraus, who have become very special people in my life. Marrisa and Eric's patience and understanding is the reason there is *Dr. Bruce Lowell's Fat Percentage Finder.*

CONTENTS

READ THIS FIRST:
HOW THIS BOOK ORIGINATED
AND WHAT IT CAN DO FOR YOU

Fat has become one of the greatest health risks known to man. Our fast-food society has borne witness to the rise of levels of dietary fat to the point where virtually all health-conscious Americans are actively trying to eliminate this potential killer from their refrigerators and cupboards.

I first became interested in the problem of eating high-fat foods before I knew it was a problem at all. I was obese. My entire family was obese. We believed that our obesity was due to the overconsumption of sweets, especially cakes and candies. We went on all kinds of diets, would lose weight, and then gain it right back.

When I completed college, I pursued my dream of becoming a doctor. I attended medical school in Belgium: the land of waffles, chocolate, and french fries with mayonnaise. It wasn't long before I realized that Europeans, as a rule, are not overweight. In medical school, I attempted to learn why my European friends could eat so much wonderful food and stay slim. After much study, I eventually realized that Europeans eat small portions and balance their consumption of dietary fat with non-fat items. I learned this technique and lost 50 pounds.

When I returned to the United States to complete my residency in Internal Medicine, I gained back the weight I had lost in Europe. I became increasingly interested in nutrition and started reading as many books as I could find on the topic. Those deadly sweets, I realized, were actually high-fat foods. I therefore learned that the problem was not consumption of too much dietary sugar, as we were always led to believe, but consumption of too much dietary fat! I wasted no time in cutting fat from my diet and balancing my favorite foods with non-fat ones. Once and for all, I lost my excess weight!

In the hospital where I was doing my residency, I had become the expert on diet. Every overweight hospital employee wanted my advice. When I informed my colleagues of my belief in the importance of nutrition, the response was always the same: Stick to medicine! Fortunately, I didn't listen.

Following my residency, I went into private practice in Internal Medicine. As my practice grew, so did my desire to treat nutritional illnesses. An opportunity to do just that presented itself when a colleague from Boston asked me to establish the first weight-management program in our area using up-to-date techniques, including low calorie diets, nutritional counselling, and behavior modification. I started this practice with my wife, Diane, who is a registered nurse. Our program became known as The Weight and Risk Management Center.

We needed a more comprehensive method of teaching people how to manage the fat in their diets, yet the actual amount of fat in food was still a mystery to us. In fact, the true fat content of most foods passed detection for decades, until:

THE 30% FAT SOLUTION

I reached a turning point in my career when I realized that no matter how much we taught our patients about calories and nutrition, they continued to eat high-fat foods. At this time, the Surgeon General and all the major health organizations were beginning to caution Americans about the dangers of dietary fat. The National Institutes of Health then issued its dietary guidelines for the country, which established a goal of consuming no more than 30% of our total calories from dietary fat. This percentage was chosen because it is attainable.

Now the question was: How do we achieve this goal? To this end, I polled patients, dieticians, and physicians. They either didn't know the meaning of "30% of total calories" or they offered solutions which were too complicated for people to understand easily. We needed help!

The NIH then stated that one way to accomplish this goal was to limit each of the foods we eat to those that contain no more than 30% fat. What a simple solution to a difficult problem! I then searched for books that listed the percentage of fat in individual foods. Surprisingly, such a book did not exist. It seemed the solution wasn't as easy as I had originally believed.

Determined to uncover the hidden fats in food, I developed the concepts you will find in *Dr. Bruce Lowell's Fat Percentage Finder.* I advised my patients to eat a majority of foods having a fat content of 30% or less. To help them, I created many of the lists found in this book. The results were astounding. People adapted easily to this new way of eating, lost weight and lowered their cholesterol. I had found the key! This easy way to limit the fat in our diet is the beginning of a new era in maintaining good health.

Dr. Bruce Lowell's Fat Percentage Finder has a simple goal: To help you comply with the 30% fat guideline established by the NIH. You will accomplish this by checking the food lists in this book and by eating foods that contain 30% or less fat. I've listed the percentage of fat in over 6000 brand-name and basic foods. I have also developed a unique chart to help you find the hidden fat in any food, even in those not listed in this guide. I call this chart "Dr. Lowell's Label Fat Percentage Finder." For those readers needing a precise method for measuring fat, I have included fat/gram requirement tables for both men and women.

Dr. Bruce Lowell's Fat Percentage Finder has two parts: The Fat Connection and The Food Lists. In The Fat Connection, we will examine the problems of excessive fat intake as well as solutions to those problems. The Food Lists simply expose the hidden fat in foods, making shopping and menu planning fun and easy.

I hope you will enjoy this book as much as I have enjoyed writing it. The 30% Fat Solution has changed many people's lives for the better, and it will do the same for you. Remember, good health is not attained by magic, fast cures, or fad diets. The 30% Fat Solution is for a lifetime.

Part One
THE FAT CONNECTION

1. EXCESSIVE DIETARY FAT:
A MAJOR HEALTH RISK

Our high-fat consumption has created a state of "overnutrition," which is linked to many health problems. By the end of Part One of *Dr. Bruce Lowell's Fat Percentage Finder,* you will understand the importance of the 30% Fat Solution and its role in promoting good health.

First, here are the problems linked to excessive fat:

OBESITY

Obesity is the result of consuming too many calories above our energy needs. Most of these excessive calories are derived from dietary fat. It takes very little energy to convert these excessive fat calories into body fat. Simply put: Fat makes us fat! Since fat likes to "hide" in the foods we eat, its detection and elimination can be difficult.

HEART AND VASCULAR DISEASE

Recent evidence has shown that excessive dietary fat is a major cause of heart and other vascular-linked diseases. The high intake of animal and tropical fats raises cholesterol levels, which in turn may lead to premature aging and the narrowing of the blood vessels. This may cause heart attack, stroke, kidney disease and other degenerative organ illnesses. We all need the 30% Fat Solution to help prevent these deadly diseases.

DIABETES

Diabetes is a major cause of suffering and premature death due to severe vascular damage. Adult onset of non-insulin dependent diabetes mellitus results from a relative lack of insulin, which is caused by increasing obesity. Insulin produced by our body acts on fat cells to control blood sugar and blood fats. As body fat increases, so does the need for additional insulin. We then reach a point at which our body cannot keep up with the amount of insulin it needs, given the increased amount of body fat. My obese diabetic patients need the 30% Fat Solution to lose weight, lower blood-fat levels, and decrease cholesterol. This may, in fact, be all they need to control their illness.

CANCER

Uterine cancer, breast cancer in the post-menopausal woman, colon cancer, and prostate cancer have all been linked to high levels of dietary fat and obesity.

Excessive amounts of hormones are stored as body fat increases. High fat-hormone levels cause prolonged stimulation of hormone-receptive body organs such as the prostate, breast, and female reproductive organs. It is believed that this stimulation may be the cause of some cancers. Cancer of the colon, for example, is common in societies where excessive fat is consumed. Dietary fat has a slowing effect on intestinal mobility, causing constipation, which in turn allows the carcinogens found in the foods we eat to become stagnant in the body. This causes increased stimulation of the cells in the intestinal wall, which may induce cancer. We all need to reduce the risk of cancer, however, and the 30% Fat Solution is a simple nutritional goal that will help us do so.

GALL BLADDER DISEASE

Obesity and high fat intake both cause the bile produced by the gall bladder to form gall stones. When there is a high fat concentration in bile, the naturally dissolved contents of the gall bladder precipitate, thus forming gall stones. This may lead to gall bladder attacks and infection, which requires the surgical removal of the gall bladder. The 30% Fat Solution will reduce weight, lower the amount of fat concentration in the gall bladder, and help prevent gall stones.

ARTHRITIS

Obesity aggravates our bodies' major weight-bearing joints. Increased weight also accelerates the normal wear and tear on the spine, hips, and knees. Eating a high-fat diet can also precipitate painful gout attacks through the retention of uric acid. The 30% Fat Solution will help decrease this possibility and lessen the wear and tear on the large joints.

IMMUNE SYSTEM

Recent evidence has shown that we are more likely to succumb to illness if we consume high levels of dietary fat. Lymphocytes are natural disease fighters found in the bloodstream that kill bacteria and viruses. High dietary fat may suppress these disease-fighting lymphocytes. The 30% Fat Solution will help prevent this from occurring.

The connection of high-fat intake to illness has definitely been established. Too much fat makes us sick! We now need to learn how to limit its intake.

2. THE 30% FAT SOLUTION

As you will discover, the lists in *Dr. Bruce Lowell's Fat Percentage Finder* provide you with the percentage of fat found in the foods we eat. They help make choosing low-fat items fun and easy. First it is necessary to explain some of the difficulties in uncovering hidden fat.

Fat can hide in the label's nutritional information or in the product name. Once you fully understand the concept of hidden fat, you will never look at food the same way again!

HOW FAT HIDES IN OUR FOODS AND LABELS

Everyone on the planet knows that whole milk is high in fat. But, how about a product that is reduced in calories? First, look at the food label to see if you can spot the hidden fat. For example, let's take a look at Marie's "Lite" salad dressing. Don't be too shocked!

Marie's Lite Thousand Island Dressing

Serving size	1 Tablespoon
Servings per container	16
Calories	40
Protein	0 grams
Carbohydrates	3 grams
Fat	3 grams

To find the hidden fat in this salad dressing, we must pick apart the label. Remember, the calories and grams listed are for the portion size on the label—one tablespoon. In order for us to see how much fat is actually in this dressing we must convert the grams into calories to expose the fat-calorie content.

We can convert grams into calories with the following formulas:

1 gram of protein = 4 calories
1 gram of carbohydrate = 4 calories
1 gram of fat = 9 calories

Going back to the Marie's Lite label: 1 Tablespoon of salad dressing = 40 calories, which breaks down as follows:

0 grams of protein	× 4 calories/gram =	0 calories
3 grams of carbohydrates	× 4 calories/gram =	12 calories
3 grams of fat	× 9 calories/gram =	27 calories
Total		39 calories

You can see that twice the amount of calories come from fat than from protein and carbohydrates in this "lite" salad dressing. By converting the label with our formula, we were able to expose the hidden fat—all 27 calories of it!

To determine the percentage of fat in Marie's Lite we simply divide the 27 fat calories that we just uncovered by the total calories per serving, which was 40. (27 ÷ 40 = .68.) You then multiply .68 by 100 to arrive at the 68% value. So we see that this "lite" salad dressing is, in fact, 68% fat!

Before *Dr. Bruce Lowell's Fat Percentage Finder,* the consumer had to use this formula to convert every label to reveal the hidden fats in foods. Fortunately, the *Fat Percentage Finder* does all the work for you!

As we have seen from the example of Marie's Lite salad dressing, fat can hide in the name of an item as well as in the nutritional information given on the label. Indeed, some confusing labeling may imply that a manufacturer has our health at interest. Let's take a look at some examples:

"Lite" or "light" is a popular word found on many labels. Although we immediately associate these words with healthy foods, they can actually refer to the color and/or weight of the item in question. For example, "lite" olive oil is light in color, but has the same amount of fat and calories as regular olive oil. The package of "lite" pretzels implies that they are low in fat, but the actual calorie amount is identical to that of the same portion of regular pretzels. Here, the "lite" simply means that each pretzel weighs less. Pretty tricky.

Health-conscious shoppers automatically tend to accept items that are labeled "low cholesterol," "cholesterol free," and "reduced calories." Do these products fit into the 30% Fat Solution? Let's take a look: Low-cholesterol, reduced-calorie mayonnaise has fewer calories than regular mayonnaise, but also has a whopping 92% fat. Regular mayonnaise has 100 calories per tablespoon and 100% fat, whereas the "reduced" variety has 50 calories per tablespoon, but is still very high in fat.

An item touted as being "97% Fat-Free" must be low in fat—or is it? The fat content of such foods as luncheon meats and dairy products is a percentage of the total weight or volume. This allows for water, which has no calories! Since the water in 99% fat-free milk accounts for the majority of its volume, we can see that it still has 25% of its calories from fat! This may be illustrated by adding water to powdered milk.

The word "dietetic" implies that a product is low in calories. Stella D'Oro Prune Pastry, for example, is labeled dietetic. Although this product has less sugar than regular Stella D'Oro Prune Pastry, it is still 40% fat.

Does "low fat" mean that a product has less than 30% fat? Government regulations stipulate that "low fat" means 40% or less. This certainly does not fit into the 30% Fat Solution, so be careful.

"Natural" products are from nature, so they must be low in fat, right? Wrong. Take a look at coconut oil: you'll never find a more natural product, yet it has the highest saturated fat content on the planet. So we can see that the term "natural" has absolutely nothing to do with fat content.

Products labeled "fat free" do fit into the 30% Fat Solution, so add them to your shopping list.

For labels that do not contain nutritional information, consult the list of ingredients usually found on the side of the package. Ingredients are listed in order of highest to lowest content. If you see fat listed as the second or third ingredient: Beware.

Your best choice is to do as I do and check the food lists in this book before shopping and scrutinize the labels in the store using the Label Fat Percentage Finder. It's fun and it's easy.

By now you should realize that eating a high-fat diet was not really your fault. It was impossible to know where all of this dietary fat was coming from! It was so easy to assume that all low-cholesterol, lite, reduced-calorie, dietetic, fat-free, and natural products were good for us. Now that we have exposed the problem of hidden fat, we are ready to embark upon the 30% Fat Solution.

PERCENTAGE OF FAT IN FOOD
The more than 6000 food entries, with their fat percentages, listed in this book will help you accomplish the 30% Fat Solution. The lists are categorized based upon the way we eat, and foods are listed under their brand and basic names. The beginning of each group displays the fat range as well as the average fat for all the foods in that group. Fat grams are listed as well as the calories for each food. *The single most important listing, however, is percentage of fat.* All the hidden fats are exposed, leaving no doubt whether or not any given food fits into the 30% Fat Solution.

For example, take a look at the Cookie Section on pages 39–42. Find one of your favorite cookies and examine its percentage of fat. Now do some comparing. Vanilla Wafers are 21% fat as compared to S'more Girl Scout Cookies, which are 56% fat. To maintain the 30% Fat Solution, simply choose the Vanilla Wafers. In the fish section, you can see that fried bass tops the limit with 40% fat, whereas baked bass is a desirable 18% fat. It's amazing to see how the once-difficult task of eating a low-fat diet has now become easy and fun!

KNOWING FAT-GRAM REQUIREMENTS
For the readers who need to be very exact in their pursuit of the 30% Fat Solution, the Requirement Tables, showing both calories and fat grams, will be a valuable aide in selecting low-fat foods.

If you are overweight, diabetic, or suffer from serious cholesterol-metabolism problems, you should use this section as an extra aide. Tables I and II provide the exact amounts of grams of fat needed per day based on your weight and caloric requirements.

I will explain how to use this information in the "How to Use This Book" section. First, however, it is important to understand some key facts about fats and other nutrients.

3. IMPORTANT NUTRITIONAL FACTS

Saturated, polyunsaturated, and monosaturated are the three different types of fats found in food. Most fats are mixtures of all three types but are grouped according to the most prevalent.

Saturated Fat

This fat stays solid at room temperature. Saturated fats are inexpensive, have a long shelf life and don't break down during frying. Saturated fats are favorites in the fast-food industry and cause our cholesterol levels to rise. Fats included in this category are animal fats such as lard, butter, and beef fat as well as tropical fats such as coconut and palm oil.

Polyunsaturated Fat

This fat is liquid at room temperature and is derived from plant oils such as corn, sunflower, and safflower. This fat has been linked to free radical formation, which leads to vascular breakdown and ultimately causes cancer.

Monosaturated Fat

This fat is liquid at room temperature and clouds at lower temperatures. Olive oil is a common example of a monosaturated fat. This fat is not linked to the elevation of cholesterol, but does promote obesity.

Hydrogenation

This is a process in which a less saturated fat is made more saturated. Hydrogenated fats are found in many snack foods. Hydrogenated corn oil is an example of a polyunsaturated fat being made into a saturated fat. Deep-fat frying also aids in the saturation process.

Turn to the "Fats and Oils" section of your Fat Finder for a complete classification of fats.

CHOLESTEROL FACTS

Limiting dietary fat will automatically reduce cholesterol intake. Be careful, though, for it isn't enough simply to eat foods that do not contain cholesterol to comply with the 30% Fat Solution. Tropical oils do not contain cholesterol but have the highest amount of saturated fat on the planet! Tropical oils also induce the liver to manufacture cholesterol carriers called "bad cholesterol" or LDL. This will cause the blood levels of cholesterol to elevate. So, even though animal fats are the only fats that actually contain cholesterol, we can see that other fats like tropical oils encourage the body to make cholesterol on its own.

I have two laws that will simplify your cholesterol control:

Lowell's Law #1

Any food that needs to be caught or comes from a source that needs to be caught contains varying amounts of cholesterol. (Meat, dairy, poultry, and fish.)

Lowell's Law #2

Any food that contains an ingredient that sounds like it comes from a place you'd like to go on vacation will raise your cholesterol level. (Palm, coconut, and palm kernel oil.)

The cholesterol in our bloodstream is measured in three ways: LDL cholesterol, HDL cholesterol, and total cholesterol. LDL or "bad cholesterol" is the portion of the total cholesterol that promotes vascular disease. LDL cholesterol is increased by consuming foods containing cholesterol and saturated fats. Our LDL should not exceed 130 mg per 100 cc of blood (%). LDL has an "L" in it, meaning it should be low. HDL, or "good cholesterol" is the portion of total cholesterol that is advantageous in that it helps to rid the body of plaque-forming cholesterol associated with hardening of the arteries. HDL cholesterol is increased by exercise and by following a low-fat diet. HDL cholesterol should be above 45 mg%. HDL has an "H" in it, meaning it should be high. Our total cholesterol level, representing the summation of all the cholesterol found in the bloodstream, should not exceed 200 mg%.

PROTEIN FACTS

The average adult needs only 4 to 6 ounces of protein a day. When eaten in smaller amounts, protein can actually lower fat and cholesterol consumption.

Protein foods, especially meat products, are very high in hidden saturated fat. Eating smaller amounts will therefore lower the amount of fat consumed. Eggs, poultry, meat, and fish are excellent sources of protein. *Dr. Bruce Lowell's Fat Percentage Finder* will help you to choose delicious low-fat foods that will comply with the 30% Fat Solution.

CARBOHYDRATE FACTS

Carbohydrates are a major source of energy, fiber, vitamins, and minerals. The more carbohydrates we eat, the more of these elements naturally enter into our diet. A diet high in complex carbohydrates requires more metabolic energy. Thus, more food may be eaten.

There are two kinds of carbohydrates:

Simple Carbohydrates

These are foods that contain large amounts of simple sugars, which dissolve easily or are in liquid form. Examples include fruit juice, syrup, and table sugar. Simple carbohydrates are utilized for quick energy and should be avoided in large quantities by those with diabetes. Simple sugars all have endings of "ose," as in fructose, sucrose and lactose.

Complex Carbohydrates

Complex carbohydrates do not become liquid when water is added. Starches, fruits, grains, vegetables, and beans are all examples of complex carbohydrates. They are excellent sources of energy, fiber, vitamins, and minerals. Highly colored complex carbohydrates such as peppers and broccoli contain beta carotene—a natural anti-cancer element. It takes more metabolic energy to break down complex carbohydrates than fat or simple carbohydrates, thus they help prevent obesity.

FIBER AND MINERALS

Fiber is plentiful in fruits, vegetables, beans, and grains. Many studies show that fiber may help lower cholesterol levels. Fiber also helps the intestinal movement of food, which may prevent stagnation of carcinogens, thus having an anti-cancer effect. Fiber also assists in the prevention of constipation and spastic-colon disorders. A diet low in fat and high in complex carbohydrates will supply the necessary fiber and minerals we all need to maintain good health.

SALT

Americans consume an overabundance of salt. The normal American diet has approximately 4 grams of salt a day. The American Heart Association recommends no more than 2 grams per day. A high-salt diet will aggravate high blood pressure and cause water retention. Salt has no caloric value. Since most high-fat foods are also high in salt, the 30% Fat Solution will help you to cut your salt intake.

In this first section we have covered the 30% Fat Solution, the Fat Connection, and Nutritional Facts. In the next section you will learn how to use this unique book.

4. HOW TO USE THIS BOOK

This section explains the organization and use of the Tables, Food Charts, and Label Fat Percentage Finder.

THE MALE AND FEMALE TABLES

These tables—one for men and one for women—are for individuals who have a medical problem such as high cholesterol, obesity, anorexia, or diabetes that requires special attention to the consumption of fat grams and calories. If you do not need this extra help, skip this section and go to "Dr. Lowell's Label Fat Percentage Finder" on page 29.

Table I
Female Daily Consumption of Calories and Maximum Fat Grams to Attain and Maintain Desired Weight.

Table II
Male Daily Consumption of Calories and Maximum Fat Grams to Attain and Maintain Desired Weight.

These tables provide the total number of calories and fat grams men and women age twenty to fifty-five are required to eat to achieve the 30% Fat Solution. Calories and fat grams are matched to body weights. Fat grams are calculated from the total calories to provide no more than 30% of daily calories from fat.

To help you understand these tables, let's take a look at three of my patients: Mary wants to maintain her weight; Jane wants to lose weight; and Bob wants to gain weight.

Mary is fifty years old, weighs 100 pounds, and has suffered a recent heart attack. She must be careful to eat no more than 30% fat in her diet. Mary has high cholesterol levels and was a chain smoker. She has tried numerous cholesterol-lowering drugs but has never attempted to lower her dietary fat intake. She is now ready to change to a low-fat lifestyle by accepting the 30% Fat Solution.

First, Mary looks at Table I on page 27 and finds her present weight of 100 pounds:

WEIGHT	CALORIES/DAY	FAT GRAM/DAY
100	1100	37

At 100 pounds, Mary should eat a total of 1100 calories a day and no more than 37 grams of fat to maintain her weight and achieve healthy eating habits. Thirty-seven grams of fat equals 330 calories. Therefore, of the 1100 calories, approximately 30% is fat.

Jane weighs 140 pounds, 20 pounds overweight. She has elevated blood sugar and a family history of diabetes. Jane wants to lose weight by healthy eating. She has tried many weight-loss programs, but has always gained weight back after dieting. In order for Jane to attain her desired weight, she must follow the 30% Fat Solution.

Jane looks at Table I on page 27 and locates her desired weight of 109 pounds:

WEIGHT	CALORIES/DAY	FAT GRAMS/DAY
109	1200	40

Jane will now eat at her desired weight range according to the low-fat guidelines. She will use the percentage of fat from the food lists to help make low-fat choices. This new eating pattern will insure that she will maintain her weight once she attains it. Jane will never have to diet again.

Our next patient is Bob—a special case. Bob weighs 167 pounds and is slightly underweight. Bob would like to gain weight before he starts a new job. His goal is 175 pounds. Bob is very health-conscious and decides to target a one pound weight gain per week over several weeks. One pound of body fat is equal to 3500 calories. If Bob adds 500 calories a day for one week he will then gain the one pound of fat: 7 days $\times$ 500 cal/day = 3500 calories.

Bob finds 167 pounds on Table II on page 28:

WEIGHT	CALORIES/DAY	FAT GRAMS/DAY
167	2000	67

Bob will then add 500 calories a day: 2000 calories
+ 500 calories
2500 calories

Bob then locates 2500 calories on Table II:

WEIGHT	CALORIES/DAY	FAT GRAMS/DAY
208	2500	80

Bob will only eat at this level until he attains his desired weight of 175 pounds. At that point, he will find his new weight on Table II and eat accordingly.

Mary, Jane, and Bob illustrate just a few of the many ways in which the reader may use these tables. Remember, these tables are for people with specific requirements and aren't necessary for the majority who wish to achieve the 30% Fat Solution.

DR. LOWELL'S LABEL FAT PERCENTAGE FINDER

I don't often go food shopping, but when I do I am usually overwhelmed by the endless number of new products that compete for our hard-earned money and precious calories. Since I can't update this book every week to keep up with the introduction of new products, I did the next best thing and created a simple chart that converts calories and grams into percentages of fat. This valuable chart has come to be known as "Dr. Lowell's Label Fat Percentage Finder" and will give you the percentage of fat in any food as long as it has a nutritional label that lists calories and grams of fat.

I was in the supermarket the other day and came upon a new product: Bruce's Lite Microwave Popcorn. I love popcorn, and since it had such an appealing name and claimed to be "lite," I had to have it! Let's take a look:

Bruce's Lite Microwave Popcorn

Nutrition Information Per Serving
Serving Size   3 Cups
Servings Per Bag   5
Calories   100 (value to be used)
Protein   0 gram
Carbohydrates   14 grams
Fat Total   5 grams (value to be used)
Saturated   4 grams
Non-Saturated   1 gram
Cholesterol   0 mg.
Sodium   170 mg.

Fortunately, I had my Label Fat Percentage Finder with me. Take a look at yours (page 29) and follow along. First, find 100 calories on the top line of the chart. Then find 5 fat grams along the left side of the chart. Draw a line connecting the calories on the top to the fat grams on the side. The point where these two lines meet is the percentage of fat.

Bruce's Lite Popcorn has 45% fat. Oh, no: This isn't a very good choice! Once again, we see a "lite" product that is anything but and that doesn't comply with the 30% Fat Solution. "Dr. Lowell's Label Fat Percentage Finder" will be your best friend in the grocery store. A "take-along" version is provided in the back of the book; simply cut it out along the black line. Like the man says: "Don't leave home without it!"

THE FAT FINDER'S FOOD LISTS

The Food Lists are your keys to achieving the 30% Fat Solution. They are arranged for either quick reference or for in-depth planning. Notice that the percentage of fat is given in the right-hand column where it is easy to see. How do your favorite foods stack up?

Over 6000 foods are listed including both low- and high-fat items. The foods have been grouped into common eating categories such as "Desserts," "Breakfast Foods," and "Fats and Oils." A special section on diet aides lists both over-the-counter and medically supervised products.

The lists are user-friendly. If you don't find a food on one list, the book will guide you to another area. The fast-food selections are quite up-to-date. We all worry about eating in fast-food restaurants, but *Dr. Bruce Lowell's Fat Percentage Finder* will not only help you select the food you eat, but will also assist in the selection of a restaurant.

Please keep the Label Fat Percentage Finder in mind as we go on to the Food Lists.

ORDER OF FOOD ENTRIES

The foods on the lists are categorized into major groups of similar foods. Examples are: Baked Goods, Beans, Beverages, and Breakfast Foods. All are listed alphabetically.

Each major section is then broken down into similar groups of foods. In the Baked Goods section, for example, you will find Bagels, Buns, and Rolls in one group. I have organized the Fat Percentage Finder in this manner for several reasons: First, it provides an easy way to find foods in the order that we normally eat them. Secondly, it allows comparison of major groupings of foods to determine which group is higher in fat. Thirdly, it allows for comparison shopping of foods within the same group.

FAT RANGE

The Fat Range calculation is found at the beginning of each food grouping and represents the percentage of fat in that group from lowest to highest. When you select a food from that group, the Fat Range will help you find the lower-fat choice whenever possible.

Let's take a look at a common food group: Sandwiches. You're in your favorite deli at lunchtime and you're dying for a sandwich. Turning to the sandwich section of the Fat Finder you see that the Fat Range of that group is 20%–73%. A turkey sandwich without mayonnaise has only 23% fat—well within the 30% Fat Solution!

AVERAGE FAT

Under a food group's Fat Range you will also discover the Average Fat Percentage for all the foods listed in that group. This makes it easy to identify high- and low-fat groups. For example, you feel like having a dessert but can't decide between a doughnut or cookies. Checking the Average Fat heading for both, you discover that doughnuts have an Average Fat of 49% whereas cookies are a more acceptable 38%. You then proceed to the cookie section where you will find selections such as Vanilla Wafers, with low fat percentages. At 21% fat, Vanilla Wafers comply with the 30% Fat Solution and taste great! Remember: Average Fat is an average of both low- and high-fat choices in a food group and should only be used as a quick reference point.

STARRED ITEMS

A star (*) appears in the far left column next to foods with a fat percentage of 30% or less. This will enable you to identify quickly low-fat choices and make grocery shopping a breeze!

PORTION COLUMN

Here and there you will find special instructions regarding portion size. The portion is the amount listed on the label by the manufacturer. Occasionally, a manufacturer will list a smaller-than-usual portion to make an item appear less caloric. Some "lite" salad dressings, for example, list a portion of one teaspoon rather than one tablespoon. The lists of abbreviations and equivalent measures used in the portion column are found on page 30.

CALORIES

Calories are listed according to portion size. When the portion changes, so does the caloric value. These values represent the latest information available and can change according to a manufacturer's modification of ingredients.

FAT GRAMS

Fat grams are listed according to portion size. Some foods in small portions only have a trace of fat and are accordingly assigned a value of 0 fat grams.

PERCENT FAT

Percent Fat is found in the far right column. Percentage of fat exposes the hidden fats in foods. This concept underlies the 30% Fat Solution. Remember: *The percentage of fat will not change even if the portion size changes.* This is your key to the 30% Fat Solution.

EXAMPLE FROM THE FOOD LIST

Let's put all these elements together and take a look at the first entry on the Food List:

BAKED GOODS

■ **BAGELS, BUNS, AND ROLLS**
  Fat Range = 0%–58%
  Average Fat = 19%

FOOD	MEASURE OR QUANTITY	CALORIES	FAT GRAMS	% FAT
*Bagel, Rye (Lenders)	1	150	1	6

1. The Fat Range for this group is 0%–58%
2. The Average Fat is 19%
3. A star (*) means 30% fat or less
4. Bagel (common name); Rye (flavor); Lender's (manufacturer)
5. The portion is one bagel
6. There are 150 calories in one bagel
7. There is one gram of fat in one bagel
8. One bagel has 6% of its calories from fat

Congratulations! You now have all the tools you need to eat according to the 30% Fat Solution!

5. MAKING THE 30% FAT SOLUTION WORK FOR YOU

Here are some practical hints that I have shared with my patients over the years:

1. Keep a food diary for one week and write down everything you eat. Then use the Fat Percentage Finder to see how many of the foods you ate were above 30% fat. Go through your kitchen cabinets and check out the percentages of fat in the food in the house. Are you eating a low-fat diet?

2. The 30% Fat Solution is for a lifetime. You have to start sometime, so do it now. Begin by choosing low-fat breakfast foods from the Fat Percentage Finder. A high-fat choice may be balanced with a low-fat choice at the next meal. Before long this will become second nature. If you have a high-fat day, simply balance it with a day of low-fat eating.

3. Scan the Food Lists before you go shopping. Snack foods are fine if you make low-fat choices. Air-popped popcorn has 0% fat but Microwave PopRite has 38% fat. Select the cuts of poultry and meat that are low in fat. Light chicken meat without skin is 26% fat. Add skin and add another 19% to make a total of 45% fat. Use the Label Fat Percentage Finder before you pick up any new product. Remember Bruce's Lite Microwave Popcorn!

4. If you have a special problem, use the Requirement Tables. Select foods that are starred. This will keep your fat content within the 30% Fat Solution.

5. Pay strict attention to portion size! A low-fat food may become a high-fat choice by increasing the portion.

6. Add new products to your Fat Percentage Finder for future reference.

7. Become a 30% Fat Solution expert. This will help you to maintain a healthy lifestyle as well as to educate your family and friends about the dangers of hidden fats. Eating a low-fat diet will help you look and feel great.

8. Remember, by eating a low-fat diet you can actually eat more foods!

RESTAURANT EATING

Many people are afraid that they will not be able to maintain the 30% Fat Solution when they eat out. The following hints will help you:

1. Carry the Fat Percentage Finder with you!

2. Check the food lists prior to entering any deli or restaurant. Knowing what to order in advance eliminates much of the anxiety.

3. Check the lists for Italian, Mexican, and Oriental foods before ordering your favorite pasta, tortilla, or chow mein.

4. When eating at a fast-food restaurant, find the low-fat choice on the Food List. At Burger King, for example, the Burger King Broiler is 38% fat as compared to the Whopper Double Cheeseburger at 51%.

5. Ask for salad dressings and sauces on the side, and use a fork instead of a spoon to put them on your food.

6. When in doubt, rely on your senses. If something looks, smells, feels, or tastes oily or greasy—it's high in fat.

7. Many restaurants now list the calories and grams of their entrees on the menu. This is a perfect opportunity to use your Label Fat Percentage Finder to make the low-fat choice.

8. Beware of so-called "diet plates," which often offer high-fat items such as tuna salad (47%) and whole milk cottage cheese (44%).

CONCLUSION

I hope that I have conveyed the importance of eating according to the 30% Fat Solution. Remember, this is not a "diet" book, but a simple guide that will help you to reduce your fat intake, maintain a healthy lifestyle, and feel good about yourself.

I have been using the 30% Fat Solution with my patients in the Lowell Metabolics Program for years and couldn't be more pleased with the results. I have seen cholesterol levels fall, weight disappear, diabetes improve, and, above all, I have delighted in the improved lifestyles and sense of general well-being of those who choose to live by the 30% Fat Solution.

The world health organizations are all correct about the 30% Fat Solution. By simply embracing a low-fat diet we can improve our health, reduce the risk of disease, and feel fantastic. *Dr. Bruce Lowell's Fat Percentage Finder* will help you to attain this all-important goal.

TABLE I
FEMALE DAILY CONSUMPTION OF CALORIES AND MAXIMUM FAT GRAMS
TO ATTAIN AND MAINTAIN DESIRED WEIGHT

WEIGHT	CALORIES/DAY	FAT GRAMS/DAY
73	800	27
91	1000	33
100	1100	37
109	1200	40
118	1300	43
127	1400	47
136	1500	50
145	1600	53
155	1700	57
164	1800	60
173	1900	63
182	2000	67
191	2100	70
200	2200	73
209	2300	77
218	2400	80
227	2500	83
236	2600	87
245	2700	90
255	2800	93
264	2900	97
273	3000	100

Weight corresponding to calorie value is for average female, aged 20 to 55

TABLE II
MALE DAILY CONSUMPTION OF CALORIES AND MAXIMUM FAT GRAMS
TO ATTAIN AND MAINTAIN DESIRED WEIGHT

WEIGHT	CALORIES/DAY	FAT GRAMS/DAY
67	800	27
83	1000	33
92	1100	37
100	1200	40
108	1300	43
117	1400	47
125	1500	50
133	1600	53
142	1700	57
150	1800	60
158	1900	63
167	2000	67
175	2100	70
183	2200	73
192	2300	77
200	2400	80
208	2500	83
217	2600	87
225	2700	90
233	2800	93
242	2900	97
250	3000	100
258	3100	103
267	3200	107
275	3300	110
283	3400	113
292	3500	117
300	3600	120
308	3700	123
317	3800	127
325	3900	130
333	4000	133

Weight corresponding to calorie value is for average males, aged 20 to 55

DR. LOWELL'S LABEL FAT PERCENTAGE FINDER

							CALORIES										
	Grams	50	75	100	125	150	175	200	225	250	275	300	325	350	375	400	
F	1	18	12	9	7	6	5	4	4	4	3	3	3	3	2	2	
A	2	36	24	18	14	12	10	9	8	7	7	6	6	5	5	4	
T	3	54	36	27	22	18	15	14	12	11	10	9	8	8	7	7	
	4	72	48	36	29	24	21	18	16	14	13	12	11	10	10	9	
	5	90	60	45	36	30	26	22	20	18	16	15	14	13	12	11	
G	6	100	72	54	43	36	31	27	24	22	20	18	17	15	14	14	
R	7		84	63	50	42	36	32	28	25	23	21	19	18	17	16	**P**
A	8		96	72	58	48	41	36	32	29	26	24	22	21	19	18	**E**
M	9			81	65	54	46	40	36	32	29	27	25	23	22	20	**R**
S	10			90	72	60	51	45	40	36	33	30	28	26	24	22	**C**
																	E
	11			99	79	66	57	50	44	40	36	33	30	28	26	25	**N**
	12				86	72	62	54	48	43	39	36	33	31	29	27	**T**
	13				94	78	67	58	52	47	43	39	36	33	31	29	
	14					84	72	63	56	50	46	42	39	36	34	32	**F**
	15					90	77	68	60	54	49	45	42	39	36	34	**A**
																	T
F	16					96	82	72	64	58	52	48	44	41	38	36	
A	17						87	76	68	61	56	51	47	44	41	38	
T	18						93	81	72	65	59	54	50	46	43	40	
	19						98	86	76	68	62	57	53	49	46	43	
	20							90	80	72	65	60	55	51	48	45	
G	21							94	84	76	69	63	58	54	50	47	
R	22							99	88	79	72	66	61	57	53	50	
A	23								92	83	75	69	64	59	55	52	
M	24								96	86	79	72	66	62	58	54	
S	25								100	90	82	75	69	64	60	56	
	26									94	85	78	72	67	62	58	
	27									97	88	81	75	69	65	61	
	28									100	92	84	78	72	67	63	
	29										95	87	80	75	70	65	
	30										98	90	83	77	72	68	

USING THE FAT FINDER
1. Calories from nutritional panel are found on top line
2. Fat Grams from nutritional panel are found along the side
3. Join a straight line from calories to fat grams to find percent fat
4. *PICK FOODS THAT ARE 30% FAT OR LESS*
5. Take this copy when shopping
6. EXAMPLE: 150 CALORIES WITH 5 GRAMS FAT = 30% FAT

CONVERSION TABLES

Fluid

1 t	= 1/3 T	= 1/6 fl oz
3 t	= 1 T	= 1/2 fl oz
2 T	= 1/8 cup	= 1 fl oz
4 T	= 1/4 cup	= 2 fl oz
8 T	= 1/2 cup	= 4 fl oz
12 T	= 3/4 cup	= 6 fl oz
14 T	= 7/8 cup	= 7 fl oz
16 T	= 1 cup	= 8 fl oz
1 pint	= 2 cups	= 16 fl oz
1 quart	= 2 pints	= 32 fl oz
1 gallon	= 4 quarts	= 128 fl oz

Weight

1 weighed ounce	= 28.35 grams
16 weighed ounces	= 1 pound
1 pound	= 454 grams
1 kilogram	= 2.21 pounds
1 kilogram	= 1000 grams

Human Energy Conversions

1 gram of carbohydrate	= 4 Calories
1 gram of protein	= 4 Calories
1 gram of fat	= 9 Calories
1 gram of alcohol	= 7 Calories
1 pound of body fat	= 3500 Calories

ABBREVIATIONS

cnd	canned
env	envelope
pkg	package
fl oz	fluid ounce
froz	frozen
gr	gram
oz	ounce
%	percent
Lb	pound
pt	pint
sl	slice
T	tablespoon
t	teaspoon

Part Two
THE FOOD LISTS

1. BAKED GOODS

■ BAGELS, BUNS, AND ROLLS
Fat Range = 8% to 58%
Average Fat = 19%

FOOD	MEASURE OR QUANTITY	CALORIES	FAT GRAMS	% FAT
Bagel:				
*Cinnamon Raisin (Sara Lee)	1	240	2	8
Egg:				
*(Sara Lee)	1	240	2	8
*(Lender's)	1	150	1	6
*Garlic (Lender's)	1	160	1	6
Onion:				
*(Sara Lee)	1	220	1	4
*(Lender's)	1	160	1	6
Plain:				
*(Bagel Shop)	1 oz	70	0	0
*(Bagel Shop)	4 oz	280	1	3
*(Lender's)	1	150	1	6
*(Sara Lee)	1	230	1	4
Poppy Seed:				
*(Lender's)	1	150	1	6
*(Sara Lee)	1	230	1	4
*Pumpernickel (Lender's)	1	160	1	6
*Raisin and Honey (Lender's)	1	200	1	4
*Rye (Lender's)	1	150	1	6
*Sesame Seed (Lender's)	1	160	1	6
Croissants				
(See Breakfast Foods)				
Buns:				
Frankfurter:				
*(Pepperidge Farm)	1	140	3	19
*(Roman Meal)	1	104	2	17
*(Store Brand)	1	120	3	22
*(Wonder)	1	120	3	22
Hamburger:				
*(Pepperidge Farm)	1	130	3	21
*(Roman Meal)	1	113	2	16
*(Store Brand)	1	120	3	22
*(Wonder)	1	120	3	22
Rolls:				
*Brown and Serve (Pepperidge Farm)	1	100	1	9
Butter (Pepperidge Farm)	1	110	6	49
*Buttermilk (Wonder)	2	170	5	26
Dinner:				
Butterflake (Pillsbury)	1	110	4	33
*Country White (Pillsbury)	1	100	1	9
Crescent (Pillsbury)	2	200	11	50
*Parkerhouse (Pillsbury)	2	150	3	18
*(Pepperidge Farm)	1	60	2	30
*(Wonder)	2	200	4	18

FOOD	MEASURE OR QUANTITY	CALORIES	FAT GRAMS	% FAT
*Finger (Pepperidge Farm)	1	60	2	30
French:				
*(Pepperidge Farm)	1	240	2	8
*(Wonder)	2	150	5	30
*Gem Style (Wonder)	2	170	5	26
Golden Twist				
(Pepperidge Farm)	1	110	6	49
*Half and Half (Wonder)	2	160	5	28
*Home Baked (Wonder)	2	170	5	26
*Kaiser (Wonder)	1	460	8	16
*Mix (Pillsbury)	2	200	4	18
Old Fashioned (Pillsbury)	1	50	2	36
*Parker House				
(Pepperidge Farm)	1	30	1	30
Sandwich:				
*Cracked Wheat				
(Pepperidge Farm)	1	150	3	18
*Mustard Bran				
(Pepperidge Farm)	1	130	3	21
*Poppy Seed				
(Pepperidge Farm)	1	130	3	21
*Sesame Seed				
(Pepperidge Farm)	1	130	3	21
*Soft Family Style				
(Pepperidge Farm)	1	100	2	18
*Sourdough (Pillsbury)	1	100	1	9
*Wheat Loaf (Pillsbury)	1	80	2	22

■ BISCUITS

Fat Range = 10% to 50%
Average Fat = 33%

FOOD	MEASURE OR QUANTITY	CALORIES	FAT GRAMS	% FAT
Baking Powder:				
(1869 Brand)	2	200	10	45
(Pillsbury)	2	110	5	41
*Butter (Pillsbury)	2	100	2	18
Butter Flavor (Continental)	2	190	8	38
Buttermilk:				
Big Country (Pillsbury)	2	200	8	36
Deluxe (Pillsbury)	2	280	15	48
*Extra Lights (Pillsbury)	2	100	3	27
*Extra Rich (Hungry Jack)	2	110	3	25
Fluffy (Hungry Jack)	2	180	8	40
*Heat 'n Eat (Pillsbury)	2	170	5	26
*(Pillsbury)	2	100	2	18
*(Weight Watchers)	2	90	1	10
Buttertastin:				
(1869 Brand)	2	200	10	45
Big Country (Pillsbury)	2	190	8	38
(Hungry Jack)	2	180	7	35

FOOD	MEASURE OR QUANTITY	CALORIES	FAT GRAMS	% FAT
*Country (Pillsbury)	2	100	2	18
Flaky (Hungry Jack)	2	170	7	37
Good 'n Buttery (Pillsbury)	2	180	10	50
Homemade	1	100	5	45
*Homestyle (Continental)	2	100	2	18
Mountain Man (Continental)	2	190	8	38
Southern Style, Big Country (Pillsbury)	2	200	8	36
Tenderflake (Pillsbury)	2	100	5	45
Texas Style (Continental)	2	210	9	39
*Wheat (Weight Watchers)	2	90	1	10

■ **BREADS**
Fat Range = 0% to 34%
Average Fat = 11%

FOOD	MEASURE OR QUANTITY	CALORIES	FAT GRAMS	% FAT
Bagel (See Bagels, Buns, and Rolls)				
Bran, Honey:				
*(Pepperidge Farm)	1	95	1	9
*(Roman Meal Light)	1	40	0	0
*Bran'nola Original (Arnold)	1	70	1	13
Bread Stick:				
*Italian (Arnold)	1	90	1	10
*Mix (Pillsbury)	1	100	3	27
*(Store Brand)	1	35	0	0
Cinnamon Raisin:				
*(Pepperidge Farm)	1	85	2	21
*(Store Brand)	1	80	1	11
Cornbread:				
*(Aunt Jemima)	1	200	6	27
*(Store Brand)	1	180	6	30
French:				
*Mix (Pillsbury)	1	60	1	15
*(Store Brand)	1	80	1	11
*Fruit and Nut, Mix (Pillsbury)	1	160	4	22
Garlic (Arnold)	1	80	3	34
Italian:				
*(Arnold)	1	70	1	13
*(Arnold Light)	1	40	0	0
*Mix (Pillsbury)	1	60	0	0
*(Store Brand)	1	80	1	11
*Thick Slice (Arnold)	1	70	1	13
*Multigrain, Very Thin (Pepperidge Farm)	1	40	0	0
Oat:				
*Bran'nola (Arnold)	1	90	2	20
*Milk & Honey (Arnold)	1	60	1	15
*(Roman Meal)	1	70	1	13

FOOD	MEASURE OR QUANTITY	CALORIES	FAT GRAMS	% FAT
Oatmeal:				
*(Arnold Light)	1	40	0	0
*(Pepperidge Farm)	1	70	2	26
Pita:				
*(Meditteranean)	2-½ oz	160	0	0
*(Sahara)	1 oz	80	1	11
*(Sahara)	2 oz	160	1	6
*(Sahara)	3 oz	240	2	8
*(Store Brand)	1	100	1	9
*Whole Wheat (Sahara)	2 oz	150	2	12
Pumpernickel:				
*(Arnold)	1	80	1	11
*Party (Pepperidge Farm)	4	70	1	13
*(Pepperidge Farm)	1	80	1	11
*(Store Brand)	1	80	1	11
*Pumpkin (Store Brand)	1	100	2	18
Raisin:				
*(Store Brand)	1	70	1	13
*Sun-Maid (Arnold)	1	70	1	13
*Tea Loaf (Arnold)	1	70	1	13
*With Cinnamon (Pepperidge Farm)	1	125	2	14
*Round Top (Roman Meal)	1	70	0	0
*Rye, Dijon (Pepperidge Farm)	1	80	1	11
*Rye, Family (Pepperidge Farm)	1	40	0	0
*Rye Jewish (Arnold)	1	80	1	11
*Rye, Levy Jewish (Arnold)	1	80	1	11
*Rye, Melba Thins (Arnold)	1	40	0	0
*Rye, Party (Pepperidge Farm)	4	60	1	15
*Rye (Store Brand)	1	70	1	13
Seven Grain:				
*Light (Roman Meal)	1	40	0	0
*Seven Grain (Roman Meal)	1	70	0	0
*Sun Grain (Roman Meal)	1	70	1	13
Wheat:				
*Bran'nola (Arnold)	1	80	1	11
*Brick Oven (Arnold)	1	90	2	20
*(Arnold)	1	60	2	30
*(Fresh Horizons)	1	50	0	0
*Golden Light (Arnold)	1	40	0	0
*Less (Arnold)	1	40	0	0
*Light (Roman Meal)	1	40	0	0
*(Pepperidge Farm)	1	85	2	21
*(Store Brand)	1	60	1	15
*(Wonder)	1	75	1	12
Wheat, Cracked:				
*(Pepperidge Farm)	1	70	1	13
*(Roman Meal)	1	70	0	0
*(Store Brand)	1	70	1	13
*Wheat Germ (Pepperidge Farm)	1	65	0	0
*Wheat, Hearty Bran'nola (Arnold)	1	90	2	20
*Wheat Mix (Pillsbury)	1	80	2	22
*Wheat, Stone Ground (Arnold)	1	50	1	18
*Wheat, Whole, Harvest (Roman Meal)	1	66	0	0

FOOD	MEASURE OR QUANTITY	CALORIES	FAT GRAMS	% FAT
*Wheatberry (Homepride)	1	75	1	12
Wheatberry, Honey:				
*(Arnold)	1	80	2	22
*(Pepperidge Farm)	1	66	1	14
*(Roman Meal)	1	66	1	14
*(Roman Meal Light)	1	40	0	0
White:				
*Brick Oven (Arnold)	1	90	1	10
*Brick Oven (Arnold)	1	60	1	15
*(Homepride)	1	75	1	12
*Less (Arnold)	1	40	0	0
*(Pepperidge Farm)	1	70	1	13
*(Roman Meal)	1	71	0	0
*(Store Brand)	1	70	1	13
*Very Thin (Arnold)	1	40	1	22
*(Wonder)	1	75	1	12
White, Light:				
*(Roman Meal)	1	40	0	0
*(Store Brand)	1	40	0	0
*(Wonder)	1	40	1	22
*White, Milk & Honey (Arnold)	1	60	1	15
White Sandwich:				
*(Pepperidge Farm)	1	65	1	14
*(Roman Meal)	1	55	0	0
*White, Toasting				
(Pepperidge Farm)	1	85	1	11
Whole Wheat:				
*(Homepride)	1	75	1	12
*(Pepperidge Farm)	1	65	2	28
*(Store Brand)	1	60	1	15
*Very Thin (Pepperidge Farm)	1	40	1	22

■ BREAD CRUMBS
  Fat Range = 0% to 8%
  Average = 2%

FOOD	MEASURE OR QUANTITY	CALORIES	FAT GRAMS	% FAT
*Corn Flake Crumbs (Kellogg's)	4 oz	110	0	0
*Herb Seasoned				
(Pepperidge Farm)	1 T	50	0	0
*Premium (Pepperidge Farm)	1 T	50	0	0
Seasoned:				
*(Contadina)	1 T	50	0	0
*(Contadina)	1 cup	430	4	8

■ BREAD STUFFINGS
PREPARED ACCORDING TO PACKAGE
Fat Range = 32% to 54%
Average Fat = 44%

FOOD	MEASURE OR QUANTITY	CALORIES	FAT GRAMS	% FAT
Americana:				
New England (Stove Top)	4 oz	180	9	45
San Francisco (Stove Top)	4 oz	170	9	48
Beef (Stove Top)	4 oz	180	9	45
Chicken:				
(Betty Crocker)	⅙ pkg	180	9	45
(Green Giant)	4 oz	170	7	37
(Stove Top)	4 oz	180	9	45
Cornbread:				
(Betty Crocker)	⅙ pkg	170	9	48
(Green Giant)	4 oz	170	6	32
(Stove Top)	4 oz	170	9	48
Croutettes (Kellogg's)	4 oz	150	9	54
Herb (Betty Crocker)	⅙ pkg	190	9	43
Mushroom (Green Giant)	4 oz	150	7	42
Rice and Butter (Stove Top)	4 oz	180	8	40
Turkey (Stove Top)	4 oz	170	9	48
Wild Rice (Green Giant)	4 oz	160	7	39

■ BROWNIES
Fat Range = 24% to 48%
Average Fat = 37%

FOOD	MEASURE OR QUANTITY	CALORIES	FAT GRAMS	% FAT
Fudge:				
*(Little Debbie)	1 pkg	240	8	30
(Pillsbury)	2″ sq	150	6	36
Double:				
(Little Debbie)	1 pkg	350	12	31
(Pillsbury)	2″ sq	160	6	34
Nut (Homemade)	1 oz	170	7	37
*Walnut (Tastycake)	1	370	10	24
Plain:				
Gourmet (Duncan Hines)	2″ sq	280	14	45
Homemade	1 oz	150	8	48
*(Lance)	1 pkg	200	6	27
Milk Chocolate (Duncan Hines)	2″ sq	160	7	39
Original (Duncan Hines)	2″ sq	160	7	39
Walnut (Pillsbury)	2″ sq	150	8	48
(Weight Watchers)	1	100	4	36

■ COOKIES

Fat Range = 0% to 64%
Average Fat = 38%

FOOD	MEASURE OR QUANTITY	CALORIES	FAT GRAMS	% FAT
Almond:				
Supreme (Pepperidge Farm)	2	140	10	64
*Toast (Stella D'Oro)	2	112	2	16
Windmill (Nabisco)	3	140	5	32
Aloha (LU)	2	150	10	60
***Amaretti** (Stella D'Oro)	2	60	2	30
Angel Bars (Stella D'Oro)	2	140	10	64
***Angel Puffs** (Stella D'Oro)	2	26	0	0
Angel Wings (Stella D'Oro)	2	145	10	62
Angelica Goodies (Stella D'Oro)	1	100	4	36
Animal Crackers:				
*Barnum (Nabisco)	11	130	4	28
*(FFV)	9	110	3	25
*(Store Brand)	10	130	4	28
*(Sunshine)	15	130	3	21
Anisette:				
*Sponge (Stella D'Oro)	2	100	1	9
*Toast (Stella D'Oro)	2	90	0	0
Apple:				
Crisps (Nabisco)	3	150	6	36
*Newtons (Nabisco)	2	110	2	16
*Nut Bar (Pepperidge Farm)	1	170	5	26
Pastry, Diet (Stella D'Oro)	1	90	4	40
Applesauce Raisin (Nabisco)	2	140	8	51
Apricot–Raspberry				
(Pepperidge Farm)	3	150	6	36
***Arrowroot** (Nabisco)	6	130	4	28
Barre Chocolate (LU)	2	130	6	42
Blueberry:				
*Bar (Pepperidge Farm)	1	170	3	16
*Newton (Nabisco)	1	90	1	10
Bordeaux (Pepperidge Farm)	3	110	5	41
Breakfast Treats (Stella D'Oro)	1	100	4	36
Brown Edge:				
(Nabisco)	5	140	6	39
Sandwich (Nabisco)	2	160	8	45
Brownie Chocolate Nut				
(Pepperidge Farm)	3	170	10	53
Brussels (Pepperidge Farm)	3	160	8	45
Brussels Mint (Pepperidge Farm)	3	200	10	45
Butter Cookie:				
(Nabisco)	6	140	5	32
(Pepperidge Farm)	3	140	6	39
Cabana Cremes				
(Girl Scout Cookie)	1	60	3	45
Cameo Sandwich Cream				
(Nabisco)	2	140	5	32
Cappuccino (Pepperidge Farm)	3	160	6	34
Caramel Patties (FFV)	2	150	7	42
***Cherry Newton** (Nabisco)	1	90	1	10

FOOD	MEASURE OR QUANTITY	CALORIES	FAT GRAMS	% FAT
Chessman (Pepperidge Farm)	3	130	6	42
Chinese Dessert (Stella D'Oro)	1	170	9	48
Chocolate:				
Chunk Pecan				
(Pepperidge Farm)	2	130	7	48
Grahams (Nabisco)	3	170	8	42
Margarite (Stella D'Oro)	1	70	3	39
Peanut Bar (Nabisco)	2	190	10	47
*Snaps (Nabisco)	6	120	4	30
Chocolate Chip:				
(Archway)	2	120	6	45
(Frookies)	1	45	2	40
(Pepperidge Farm)	3	150	8	48
Almost Home (Nabisco)	2	130	5	35
Chip-a-Roos (Sunshine)	2	130	7	48
Chips Ahoy (Nabisco)	3	160	6	34
Chips Chocolate (LU)	2	160	10	56
Chips Deluxe (Keebler)	1	90	4	40
Chips 'n Middles (Sunshine)	2	140	6	39
Chocolate (Nabisco)	3	160	7	39
Fudge, Almost Home (Nabisco)	2	160	7	39
Macaroon (Nabisco)	1	210	10	43
Chocolu (LU)	2	110	6	49
Cinnamon Raisin, Almost Home				
(Nabisco)	2	140	7	45
Coconut:				
Bars (Nabisco)	3	130	6	42
Chocolate Chip (Nabisco)	2	150	8	48
Dietetic (Stella D'Oro)	2	100	4	36
Macaroon Bar				
(Pepperidge Farm)	1	210	11	47
Marrons (Stella D'Oro)	1	60	4	60
Como Delight (Stella D'Oro)	1	140	7	45
Craquelin (LU)	2	110	6	49
Creme Wafer Sticks (Nabisco)	3	140	7	45
***Crokine** (LU)	4	40	0	0
Custard Cup (Sunshine)	2	130	6	42
Date Nut:				
Bar (Pepperidge Farm)	1	190	7	33
Granola (Pepperidge Farm)	3	160	9	51
Do-Si-Dos (Girl Scout Cookies)	1	50	2	36
***Egg Biscuits, Dietetic**				
(Stella D'Oro)	2	80	2	22
Euphrates (LU)	2	40	2	45
Fig Bar:				
*(Keebler)	1	70	1	13
*(Nabisco)	2	120	2	15
***Fig Newton** (Nabisco)	2	120	2	15
Fortune Cookie				
(Chinese Restaurant)	1	60	3	45
***Fruit Slices** (Stella D'Oro)	1	60	2	30
Fudge:				
Covered Grahams (Keebler)	2	80	4	45
Cremes (Keebler)	2	120	6	45
Stripes (Keebler)	2	100	6	54

FOOD	MEASURE OR QUANTITY	CALORIES	FAT GRAMS	% FAT
Gaufrettes (LU)	2	85	4	42
Geneva (Pepperidge Farm)	3	170	10	53
Giggles:				
(Keebler)	2	140	6	39
Vanilla (Nabisco)	2	140	6	39
*Ginger Snaps (Nabisco)	4	120	3	22
Gingerman (Pepperidge Farm)	3	100	4	36
*Graham Crackers (Nabisco)	4	120	3	22
Hazelnut (Pepperidge Farm)	3	170	9	48
Jelly Tarts (FFV)	2	115	4	31
Kettle (Nabisco)	4	140	5	32
*Kichel, Dietetic (Stella D'Oro)	1	8	0	0
*Lady Fingers (Nabisco)	2	102	3	26
Lemon Nutcrunch				
(Pepperidge Farm)	3	170	10	53
Lido (Pepperidge Farm)	2	190	11	52
Lorna Doone (Nabisco)	4	160	8	45
Mallomars:				
(FFV)	2	130	6	42
(Nabisco)	2	120	5	38
Mandarin Orange (Frookies)	1	45	2	40
Marie Lu (LU)	2	110	4	33
Marseilles Assortment				
(Pepperidge Farm)	2	90	5	50
Marshmallow Puffs (Nabisco)	2	170	6	32
Milano (Pepperidge Farm)	3	180	10	50
*Milk Lunch (LU)	2	70	2	26
Mint Milano (Pepperidge Farm)	3	230	13	51
Mint Sandwich (FFV)	2	160	7	39
Molasses:				
*(Archway)	1	100	2	18
*(Nabisco)	2	120	4	30
Nassau (Pepperidge Farm)	2	170	10	53
*Nilla Wafers (Nabisco)	6	130	4	28
Nutter Butter (Nabisco)	2	140	6	39
Oat Bran Fruit (Health Valley)	2	110	4	33
Oatmeal:				
*(Archway)	1	110	3	25
(Drakes)	3	190	7	33
Country Style (Sunshine)	2	110	5	41
Cream, Almost Home (Nabisco)	2	130	5	35
Cremes (Keebler)	2	160	6	34
*Date Filled (Archway)	1	100	2	18
Irish (Nabisco)	3	140	7	45
Old Fashioned (Keebler)	2	160	6	34
Oatmeal Raisin:				
Almost Home (Nabisco)	2	130	5	35
(Frookies)	1	45	2	40
(Pepperidge Farm)	3	170	8	42
Orange (Pepperidge Farm)	3	170	6	32
Orange Meal (Pepperidge Farm)	3	220	12	49
Oreo:				
(Nabisco)	3	150	7	42
Double (Nabisco)	2	140	7	45
Orleans (Nabisco)	3	90	6	60

FOOD	MEASURE OR QUANTITY	CALORIES	FAT GRAMS	% FAT
Palmito (LU)	2	100	6	54
Paris (Pepperidge Farm)	2	100	5	45
Peach-Apricot				
(Stella D'Oro)	1	100	4	36
Diet (Stella D'Oro)	1	90	4	40
Peanut Brittle	3	150	7	42
Peanut Butter:				
Almost Home (Nabisco)	2	140	7	45
Fudge (Nabisco)	3	150	7	42
Peanut Butter Sandwich (FFV)	2	170	8	42
Peanut Butter Sugar Wafer	3	140	7	45
Peanut Butter Wafer (Sunshine)	3	120	6	45
Peanut Cream (Nabisco)	4	140	7	45
*Pecan Crunch (Archway)	2	70	2	26
Pecan Sandies (Keebler)	1	80	5	56
Pecan Shortbread (Nabisco)	2	160	10	56
*Pims (LU)	2	100	2	18
Pirouettes:				
Chocolate Laced				
(Pepperidge Farm)	2	110	6	49
Plain (Pepperidge Farm)	3	110	7	57
Pitter Patter (Keebler)	1.	90	4	40
Prune Pastry, Diet (Stella D'Oro)	1	90	4	40
Rich 'n Chips (Keebler)	2	160	8	45
Roman Egg Biscuits				
(Stella D'Oro)	1	140	5	32
Royal Dainty (FFV)	2	120	6	45
Samoas (Girl Scout)	1	80	5	56
Sandwich Cream (Nabisco)	3	160	7	39
Schoks Chocolate (LU)	2	140	8	51
Sesame:				
Diet (Stella D'Oro)	2	86	4	42
Regular (Stella D'Oro)	2	100	4	36
Seven Grain Oatmeal (Frookies)	1	45	2	40
Seville, assortment				
(Pepperidge Farm)	2	110	5	41
*Social Tea (Nabisco)	6	130	4	28
Southport, Assortment				
(Pepperidge Farm)	2	150	9	54
Sugar Wafer:				
(Nabisco)	8	150	7	42
(Sunshine)	2	90	4	40
T.C. Rounds (FFV)	2	160	8	45
Tahiti (Pepperidge Farm)	2	170	10	53
*Tango (FFV)	2	160	5	28
*Tea Time (Nabisco)	4	100	3	27
Thin Mints (Girl Scout)	1	40	2	45
Tofu (Health Valley)	2	130	5	35
*Trefoils (Girl Scout)	1	30	1	30
Vanilla Margarite (Stella D'Oro)	1	70	3	39
*Vanilla Wafers (Sunshine)	6	130	3	21
Vienna Fingers (Sunshine)	2	140	6	39

■ COOKIES FROM MIX

Fat Range = 33% to 55%
Average Fat = 42%

FOOD	MEASURE OR QUANTITY	CALORIES	FAT GRAMS	% FAT
Butter (Homemade)	2	100	5	45
Chocolate Chip:				
(Duncan Hines)	2	130	5	35
(Homemade)	2	130	8	55
(Pillsbury)	3	200	10	45
Golden Sugar (Duncan Hines)	2	130	6	42
Oatmeal Raisin:				
(Duncan Hines)	2	130	6	42
(Homemade)	2	120	6	45
(Pillsbury)	3	200	8	36
Peanut Butter:				
(Duncan Hines)	2	140	7	45
(Homemade)	2	130	7	48
(Pillsbury)	2	130	5	35
Sugar:				
(Pillsbury)	3	190	7	33
X-mas (Homemade)	2	80	4	45

■ CRACKERS

Fat Range = 0% to 62%
Average Fat = 32%

FOOD	MEASURE OR QUANTITY	CALORIES	FAT GRAMS	% FAT
Bacon Thins (Nabisco)	7	70	4	51
Better Cheddars:				
(Nabisco)	11	70	4	51
'n Bacon (Nabisco)	10	70	4	51
'n Onion (Nabisco)	10	70	3	39
Better Nacho (Nabisco)	9	70	4	51
Blue Cheese (Nabisco)	10	70	4	51
Cheese Crackers with Peanut Butter (Nabisco)	1 pkg	130	6	42
Cheese Snack Sticks (Pepperidge Farm)	8	130	6	42
Cheese Tid Bits (Nabisco)	16	70	4	51
Cheez-It (Nabisco)	12	70	4	51
Chocolate Graham, Thin Bits (Keebler)	12	70	3	39
Cinnamon Graham, Thin Bits (Keebler)	12	70	3	39
Club (Keebler)	4	60	3	45
*****Cracker Meal** (Nabisco)	2 T	60	1	15
*****Crisp Bread Rye** (Wasa Brod)	1	50	1	18
*****Dietetic Matzo Thins** (Manischewitz)	1 oz	90	1	10

FOOD	MEASURE OR QUANTITY	CALORIES	FAT GRAMS	% FAT
*Egg Matzo (Manischewitz)	10	110	2	16
Escort (Nabisco)	3	80	4	45
*Fiber Crisp Bread (Ryvita)	1	20	0	0
*Fiber Snackbread (Ryvita)	1	14	0	0
Graham:				
*(Nabisco)	2	60	1	15
*Honey Maid (Nabisco)	1	60	1	15
Hearty Wheat (Pepperidge Farm)	4	100	4	36
Hi-Ho (Sunshine)	4	80	5	56
*Holland Rusk (Nabisco)	1	60	1	15
Italian, Great Crisps! (Nabisco)	9	70	4	51
*Krispy Saltine No Salt (Sunshine)	5	60	1	15
*Krispy Saltines (Sunshine)	5	60	1	15
Light Rye Crispbread:				
*(Finn)	1	35	1	26
*(Ryvita)	1	26	0	0
*(Wasa Brod)	1	30	0	0
*Lunch Milk Royal (Nabisco)	1	60	2	30
Malted Milk Peanut Butter (Nabisco)	2	70	3	39
*Matzo (Store Brand)	1	130	0	0
*Matzo, Egg (Store Brand)	1	130	0	0
*Matzo, No Salt (Store Brand)	1	130	0	0
*Matzo Sheet (Manischewitz)	1 oz	115	1	8
Melba Toast:				
*Bacon (Old London)	5	60	2	30
*Garlic (Lance)	2	30	0	0
*(Lance)	2	30	0	0
*Onion (Lance)	2	80	0	0
*Pumpernickel (Old London)	3	50	0	0
*Rounds (Old London)	5	60	2	30
*Rye (Old London)	5	50	1	18
Sesame (Lance)	2	25	1	36
*Sesame (Old London)	5	60	2	30
*(Store Brand)	1	20	0	0
Nacho Great Crisps (Nabisco)	8	70	4	51
Norwegian Crispbread:				
*(Kavli)	2	30	0	0
*Thick (Finn)	1	35	0	0
Nutty Wheat Thins (Nabisco)	7	80	5	56
*Ocean Crisps (FFV)	1	60	1	15
Onion:				
Tams (Manischewitz)	10	150	8	48
Wheat (Hain)	11	130	6	42
*Original Wheat Snack Bread (Ralston)	1	20	0	0
Oyster:				
*(Nabisco)	40	130	3	21
*(Ralston)	65	120	3	22
*(Sunshine)	32	120	4	30
*Oysterettes (Nabisco)	36	120	2	15
Parmesan American Heritage (Sunshine)	4	70	4	51
Peanut Butter and Cheese Snacks (Hain)	1	190	13	62

FOOD	MEASURE OR QUANTITY	CALORIES	FAT GRAMS	% FAT
Peanut Butter Cracker				
(Little Debbie)	1	140	7	45
***Pepato Tuscany Toast**				
(Tuscany)	2	90	2	20
***Pita Crisps** (Tuscany)	2	90	1	10
Pizza Nibs (Nabisco)	20	70	3	39
Pumpernickel Wheat (Hain)	10	130	6	42
Quackers (Nabisco)	30	75	3	36
Real Bacon Great Crisps				
(Nabisco)	9	70	4	51
Real Cheddar Nips (Nabisco)	13	70	3	39
Rice Cakes:				
*(Chico San)	1	35	0	0
*(Quaker)	1	35	0	0
Rich & Crisp (Ralston)	9	140	7	45
Ritz (Regular):				
Bits	22	80	5	56
Cheese	5	70	3	39
Lo-Salt	4	70	4	51
Regular	9	149	8	48
Round Toast (Planters)	2	140	7	45
***Rusk** (Nabisco)	1	38	1	24
***Ry Krisps** (Ralston)	4	90	0	0
***Rye Twins** (Lance)	2	30	1	30
Saltine:				
*(Ralston)	10	120	4	30
*Kosher (Rokeach)	10	120	3	22
(Lance)	4	50	2	36
*Premium (Sunshine)	5	60	2	30
*Unsalted Tops (Nabisco)	5	60	2	30
Savory Garlic Crisps (Nabisco)	8	70	3	39
***Sea Rounds** (Nabisco)	1	60	2	30
Sesame American Heritage				
(Sunshine)	4	70	4	51
Sesame and Cheese Twigs				
(Nabisco)	5	70	4	51
***Sesame Crisos** (FFV)	2	120	3	22
Sesame Meal Mates (Nabisco)	3	70	3	39
Sesame (Pepperidge Farm)	4	80	3	34
***Sesame Pita Crisps** (Tuscany)	2	96	2	19
***Sesame Twins** (Lance)	2	140	1	6
Sesame Wheat (Hain)	11	140	7	45
Snack Sticks:				
(Pepperidge Farm)	8	130	5	35
Pumpernickel				
(Pepperidge Farm)	8	130	5	35
Sesame (Pepperidge Farm)	8	130	5	35
Snack (Rokeach)	9	140	7	45
Snackers (Ralston)	8	140	7	45
Sociables (Nabisco)	6	70	3	39
Soup and Oyster Dandy				
(Nabisco)	8	70	4	51
Sour Cream & Onion Quackers				
(Nabisco)	30	75	4	48
Sour Cream & Onion Cracker				
Crisps (Nabisco)	8	70	4	51

FOOD	MEASURE OR QUANTITY	CALORIES	FAT GRAMS	% FAT
Sourdog (Hain)	11	130	5	35
Square Cheese (Planters)	1 oz	140	7	45
*Stone Ground Wheat (FFV)	4	60	1	15
*Sultana Soda (Nabisco)	4	60	1	15
Taco Nips (Nabisco)	14	70	4	51
Tams (Manischewitz):				
Garlic	10	153	8	47
Onion	10	150	8	48
Tam	10	147	8	49
Wheat	10	150	8	48
Thin Wheat Snacks (Lance)	7	80	4	45
Three Cracker Assortment				
(Pepperidge Farm)	4	100	4	36
Tid-Bit, Cheese (Nabisco)	16	70	4	51
Tiny Goldfish:				
*Pretzel (Pepperidge Farm)	45	130	4	28
Cheddar (Pepperidge Farm)	45	140	6	39
Parmesan (Pepperidge Farm)	45	140	6	39
(Pepperidge Farm)	45	140	7	45
Pizza (Pepperidge Farm)	45	140	7	45
Toasted Poppy American Club				
(Nabisco)	4	70	3	39
Toasted Peanut Butter				
Sandwich (Nabisco)	2	70	4	51
Toasted Rye (Keebler)	5	80	4	45
Toasted Sesame:				
(Keebler)	5	80	4	45
*Ry Crisp (Ryvita)	1	30	0	0
Toasted Wheat:				
(Keebler)	5	80	4	45
With Onion (Pepperidge Farm)	4	80	3	34
Town House:				
(Keebler)	5	80	5	56
(Ralston)	5	80	5	56
*Triscuit (Nabisco)	7	62	2	29
Tuc (Keebler)	3	70	4	51
Twigs (Nabisco)	7	70	4	51
*Uneeda Biscuit (Nabisco)	3	60	2	30
Vegetable Wheat (Hain)	11	80	3	34
Vegetable Thins (Nabisco)	7	70	4	51
Wasa Breakfast Crisp (Wasa)	1	54	2	33
Waverly (Nabisco)	4	70	3	39
Wheat American Heritage				
(Sunshine)	4	60	3	45
*Wheat and Rye (Hain)	11	120	4	30
Wheat Crispy Wafers				
(FFV)	6	70	3	39
Wheat Snacks (Ralston)	15	130	6	42
Wheat Thins:				
Cheese (Nabisco)	9	70	3	39
*(Lance)	2	30	1	30
(Nabisco)	8	70	3	39
Wheat Wafer:				
*(Lance)	4	60	2	30
(Sunshine)	8	80	4	45
Wheatsworth (Nabisco)	5	70	3	39

FOOD	MEASURE OR QUANTITY	CALORIES	FAT GRAMS	% FAT
*Zesta Saltine (Keebler)	5	60	2	30
*Zwieback (Nabisco)	2	60	1	15

■ DOUGHNUTS
Fat Range = 36% to 63%
Average Fat = 49%

FOOD	MEASURE OR QUANTITY	CALORIES	FAT GRAMS	% FAT
Apple Filled (Dunkin Donuts)	1	220	13	53
Bavarian Creme (Dunkin Donuts)	1	230	15	59
Cake:				
(Homemade)	2 oz	180	9	45
(Hostess)	1	115	8	63
Chocolate Covered (Hostess)	1	130	8	55
Chocolate Dipped (Tastycake)	1	180	10	50
Cinnamon:				
(Hostess)	1	110	6	49
(Tastycake)	1	200	9	40
Orange Glazed, Premium				
(Tastycake)	1	360	20	50
Honey Wheat:				
Mini (Tastycake)	1	65	3	42
Premium (Tastycake)	1	340	18	48
Jelly	3 oz	250	15	54
Krunch (Hostess)	1	100	4	36
Munchkin with Sugar				
(Dunkin Donuts)	1	70	4	51
Old Fashioned (Hostess)	1	180	10	50
Fudge Iced, Premium				
(Tastycake)	1	350	22	57
Plain (Tastycake)	1	170	9	48
Powdered Sugar:				
(Hostess)	1	115	6	47
(Tastycake)	1	200	10	45
Mini (Tastycake)	1	60	3	45
Sugar Coated, Mini (Tastycake)	1	80	5	56
Yeast (Homemade)	2 oz	180	9	45
Zeppoles (Homemade)	2 oz	180	9	45

■ MUFFINS
Fat Range = 6% to 36%
Average Fat = 22%

FOOD	MEASURE OR QUANTITY	CALORIES	FAT GRAMS	% FAT
*Apple Cinnamon, Mix (Betty Crocker)	1/12	120	4	30

FOOD	MEASURE OR QUANTITY	CALORIES	FAT GRAMS	% FAT
Blueberry:				
(Pepperidge Farm)	1	180	7	35
(Store Brand)	6 oz	720	26	32
Toast 'R Cakes (Thomas')	1	110	4	33
Bran:				
Store Brand	6 oz	700	26	33
Toast 'R Cakes (Thomas')	1	110	4	33
With Raisin (Pepperidge Farm)	1	180	7	35
***Carrot Walnut**				
(Pepperidge Farm)	1	170	4	21
***Cherry Tart** (Betty Crocker)	1/12	120	4	30
Cinnamon:				
Hearty Fruit (Sara Lee)	1	200	8	36
*Swirl (Pepperidge Farm)	1	190	6	28
Corn:				
*(Betty Crocker)	1/12	160	5	28
(Pepperidge Farm)	1	180	7	35
(Store Brand)	6 oz	700	26	33
*Toast 'R Cakes (Thomas')	1	120	4	30
English:				
*Bacon & Cheese				
(Pepperidge Farm)	1	140	2	13
*Cinnamon Apple				
(Pepperidge Farm)	1	140	2	13
*Cinnamon Chip				
(Pepperidge Farm)	1	160	3	17
*Honey Wheat (Thomas')	1	128	1	7
*(Pepperidge Farm)	1	135	1	7
*Raisin (Thomas')	1	150	1	6
*Sourdough (Pepperidge Farm)	1	140	1	6
*(Store Brand)	1	130	1	7
*(Thomas')	1	130	1	7
*Wheat (Pepperidge Farm)	1	130	1	7
*(Wonder)	1	130	1	7

■ PASTRY AND DANISH

Fat Range = 27% to 57% Fat
Average Fat = 40%

FOOD	MEASURE OR QUANTITY	CALORIES	FAT GRAMS	% FAT
Almond Danish (Pepperidge Farm)	1	240	10	37
Apple Danish:				
(Hostess)	1	360	20	50
(Pepperidge Farm)	1	180	7	35
Pipin'Hot (Pillsbury)	1	250	12	43
(Sara Lee)	1	120	6	45
Apple Fruit Square— Pepperidge Farm	1	230	12	47
Apple Streudel (Pepperidge Farm)	3 oz	240	11	41

FOOD	MEASURE OR QUANTITY	CALORIES	FAT GRAMS	% FAT
Apple Turnover:				
(Pepperidge Farm)	1	310	17	49
(Pillsbury)	1	170	8	42
Blueberry Danish				
(Pepperidge Farm)	1	200	8	36
Blueberry Fruit Squares				
(Pepperidge Farm)	1	220	11	45
Caramel and Nut Danish				
(Pillsbury)	1	280	13	42
Cheese Danish (Sara Lee)	1	130	8	55
Cherry Danish (Pepperidge Farm)	1	200	8	36
Cherry, Fruit Square				
(Pepperidge Farm)	1	230	12	47
Cherry Turnover:				
(Pepperidge Farm)	1	310	19	55
(Pillsbury)	1	170	8	42
Cinnamon Danish:				
Pipin' Hot (Pillsbury)	1	220	11	45
Cinnamon with icing (Hungry Jack)	1	140	7	45
Cinnamon with Icing (Pillsbury)	1	115	5	39
Cinnamon Raisin Danish with Icing (Pillsbury)	1	145	7	43
Honey Bun (Hostess)	1	450	27	54
Orange Danish with Icing (Pillsbury)	1	145	7	43
Pastry Sheet (Pepperidge Farm)	¼ sheet	260	17	59
Pastry Shell (Pepperidge Farm)	1	210	15	64
Peach, Turnover				
(Pepperidge Farm)	1	320	19	53
*Raspberry Danish (Hostess)	1	300	10	30

2. BEANS

■ **BEANS**
Fat Range = 0% to 54%
Average Fat = 11%

FOOD	MEASURE OR QUANTITY	CALORIES	FAT GRAMS	% FAT
*Adzuki Beans, Boiled	1 cup	300	0	0
Beets:				
*Cooked	2	30	0	0
*Whole	1 cup	60	0	0

FOOD	MEASURE OR QUANTITY	CALORIES	FAT GRAMS	% FAT
*Black Beans, Boiled	1 cup	230	1	4
*Broadbeans, Boiled	1 cup	190	1	5
*Cannellini Beans, Boiled	1 cup	180	1	5
*Chickpeas, Boiled	1 cup	270	4	13
*Cranberry Beans, Boiled	1 cup	240	1	4
*Fava Beans, Boiled	1 cup	180	1	5
*French Beans, Boiled	1 cup	230	1	4
*Garbanzo Beans, Boiled	1 cup	270	4	13
*Hyacinth Beans, Boiled	1 cup	228	1	4
Kidney Beans:				
*Red, Boiled	1 cup	225	1	4
*Royal Red, Boiled	1 cup	218	0	0
*White, Boiled	1 cup	180	1	5
*Lentils, Boiled	1 cup	230	1	4
Lima Beans:				
*Baby, Boiled	1 cup	230	1	4
*Boiled	1 cup	215	1	4
*Mothbeans, Boiled	1 cup	210	1	4
*Mung Beans, Boiled	1 cup	214	1	4
*Mungo Beans, Boiled	1 cup	190	1	5
*Navy Beans, Boiled	1 cup	260	1	3
*Pink Beans, Boiled	1 cup	250	1	4
*Pinto Beans, Boiled	1 cup	230	1	4
*Red Beans	½ cup	100	1	9
Soybeans:				
Green, Boiled	½ cup	130	6	42
Mature, Boiled	1 cup	300	15	45
Mature, Sprouted, Boiled	1 cup	80	4	45
*Miso	½ cup	290	9	28
Tofu, Raw	½ cup	100	6	54
*White Beans, Boiled	1 cup	250	1	4
Winged Beans, Boiled	1 cup	250	10	36
*Yardlong Beans, Boiled	1 cup	200	1	4
*Yellow Beans, Boiled	1 cup	250	2	7

■ BEAN DISHES

Fat Range = 0% to 59% Fat
Average Fat = 16%

FOOD	MEASURE OR QUANTITY	CALORIES	FAT GRAMS	% FAT
Baked Beans:				
*(B&M)	⅞ cup	330	8	22
*(Campbell's)	1 cup	250	4	14
*(Grandma Brown's)	1 cup	290	2	6
*Homemade	1 cup	380	12	28
*(Joan of Arc)	½ cup	100	1	9
*Baked Beans, Barbecue (B&M)	1 cup	310	6	17
*Baked Beans, Brick Oven (S&W)	½ cup	160	2	11

FOOD	MEASURE OR QUANTITY	CALORIES	FAT GRAMS	% FAT
*Baked Beans, Brown Sugar				
*(Van Camp's)	1 cup	285	5	16
Baked Beans & Franks				
(Campbell's)	1 cup	360	14	35
*Baked Beans, Homestyle				
(Campbell's)	1 cup	265	3	10
*Baked Beans, Honey (B&M)	⅞ cup	280	2	6
*Baked Beans, Maple Syrup				
(S&W)	½ cup	150	1	6
*Baked Beans, Old Fashioned				
(Campbell's)	1 cup	270	3	10
Baked Beans, Pork:				
*(Campbell's)	1 cup	240	3	11
*(Joan of Arc)	½ cup	130	1	7
*(S&W)	½ cup	130	2	14
*Baked Beans, Tomato Style				
(B&M)	⅞ cup	270	3	10
Baked Beans, Vegetarian:				
*(B&M)	1 cup	230	2	8
*(S&W)	1 cup	230	1	4
*Baked Beans, Western Style				
(Van Camp's)	1 cup	200	4	18
Barbecue Beans:				
*(Campbell's)	1 cup	250	4	14
*(S&W)	½ cup	135	1	7
*Bean Salad, Four Bean				
(Joan of Arc)	½ cup	120	0	0
*Bean Salad, Marinated (S&W)	½ cup	90	1	10
Bean Salad, Three Bean:				
*(Green Giant)	½ cup	80	1	11
*(Joan of Arc)	½ cup	90	0	0
Beanee Weenee (Van Camp's)	1 cup	326	15	41
*Burrito Mix (Del Monte)	½ cup	110	1	8
Chilee Weenee (Van Camp's)	1 cup	310	16	46
Chili Beans:				
*(Joan of Arc)	½ cup	100	1	9
*(S&W)	½ cup	130	1	7
(Van Camp's)	1 cup	352	23	59
Hummus, Homemade	1 cup	450	22	44
*Pork and Beans (Van Camp's)	1 cup	216	2	8
*Ranchero Beans (Campbell's)	1 cup	220	5	20
Refried Beans:				
*(Del Monte)	½ cup	130	2	14
*Homemade	1 cup	300	5	15
*Smoky Ranch Beans (S&W)	½ cup	130	2	14

3. BEVERAGES, ALCOHOLIC

■ ALE AND BEER
ALCOHOLIC BEVERAGES SHOULD BE LIMITED ON A LOW-FAT PLAN
Fat Range = 0%
Average Fat = 0%

FOOD	MEASURE OR QUANTITY	CALORIES	FAT GRAMS	% FAT
*Amstel Light	12 fl oz	95	0	0
*Becks	12 fl oz	143	0	0
*Black Horse	12 fl oz	160	0	0
*Blatz Ale	12 fl oz	155	0	0
*Bud Light	12 fl oz	108	0	0
*Budweiser	12 fl oz	144	0	0
*Busch	12 fl oz	144	0	0
*Bush, low alcohol	12 fl oz	112	0	0
*Champale, Malt Liquor	12 fl oz	170	0	0
*Colt 45	12 fl oz	156	0	0
*Coors	12 fl oz	141	0	0
*Coors Light	12 fl oz	105	0	0
*Michelob	12 fl oz	160	0	0
*Michelob Light	12 fl oz	134	0	0
*Miller Lite	12 fl oz	96	0	0
*Molson Light	12 fl oz	109	0	0
*Stroh's	12 fl oz	145	0	0

■ LIQUORS AND MIXED DRINKS
ALCOHOLIC BEVERAGES SHOULD BE LIMITED ON A LOW-FAT PLAN
Fat Range = 0% to 12%
Average Fat = 0%

FOOD	MEASURE OR QUANTITY	CALORIES	FAT GRAMS	% FAT
*Anisette	1 fl oz	100	0	0
*Apricot Brandy	1 fl oz	80	0	0
*Benedictine	1 fl oz	95	0	0
*Bloody Mary	5 fl oz	120	0	0
*Bourbon and Soda	5 fl oz	120	0	0
Coffee Liqueur:				
*(53 Proof)	1-½ oz	174	0	0
*(63 Proof)	1-½ oz	160	0	0
*Creme De Menthe	1-½ oz	190	0	0
*Daiquiri	3 fl oz	110	0	0
*Gin and Tonic	5 fl oz	170	0	0
Gin:				
*(90 Proof)	1 jigger	110	0	0

FOOD	MEASURE OR QUANTITY	CALORIES	FAT GRAMS	% FAT
*(94 Proof)	1 jigger	116	0	0
*(100 Proof)	1 jigger	124	0	0
*Manhattan	2 fl oz	130	0	0
*Martini	3 fl oz	170	0	0
*Pina Colada	5 fl oz	300	4	12
Rum:				
*(80 Proof)	1 jigger	100	0	0
*(94 Proof)	1 jigger	116	0	0
*(100 Proof)	1 jigger	124	0	0
*Screwdriver	7 fl oz	180	0	0
*Tequilla Sunrise	5 fl oz	200	0	0
*Tom Collins	5 fl oz	120	0	0
Vodka:				
*(94 Proof)	1 jigger	116	0	0
*(100 Proof)	1 jigger	124	0	0
*Whiskey Sour	4 fl oz	170	0	0
Whiskey:				
*(94 Proof)	1 jigger	116	0	0
*(100 Proof)	1 jigger	124	0	0

■ WINES

ALCOHOLIC BEVERAGES SHOULD BE LIMITED ON A LOW-FAT PLAN
Fat Range = 0%

FOOD	MEASURE OR QUANTITY	CALORIES	FAT GRAMS	% FAT
*Red Wine (Store Brand)	3-½ oz	75	0	0
*Sherry (Store Brand)	2 oz	90	0	0
Vermouth:				
*Dry (Store Brand)	3-½ oz	100	0	0
*Sweet (Store Brand)	3-½ oz	170	0	0
*White Wine (Store Brand)	3-½ oz	70	0	0
*Wine Cooler, Fruit Flavors				
(Store Brand)	12 fl oz	220	0	0

4. BEVERAGES, NON-ALCOHOLIC

■ CARBONATED BEVERAGES: SUGAR AND DIET

Fat Range = 0%
Average Fat = 0%

FOOD	MEASURE OR QUANTITY	CALORIES	FAT GRAMS	% FAT
Apple Slice:				
*Diet	12 fl oz	1	0	0
*Regular	12 fl oz	155	0	0
Cherry Coke:				
*Diet	12 fl oz	1	0	0
*Regular	12 fl oz	155	0	0
Cherry RC:				
*Diet	12 fl oz	1	0	0
*Regular	12 fl oz	170	0	0
***Club Soda** (Store Brand)	12 fl oz	0	0	0
Coca-Cola:				
*Classic	12 fl oz	155	0	0
*Diet	12 fl oz	1	0	0
***Cola** (Store Brand)	12 fl oz	150	0	0
***Cola, RC**	12 fl oz	170	0	0
***Cream Soda** (Store Brand)	12 fl oz	190	0	0
***Diet No-Cal, All Flavors**	12 fl oz	1	0	0
***Diet Pepsi-Light**	12 fl oz	1	0	0
Ginger Ale (Store Brand):				
*Diet	12 fl oz	1	0	0
*Regular	12 fl oz	150	0	0
***Mandarin Orange Slice**	12 fl oz	190	0	0
***Mineral Water All Types**				
(Store Brand)	12 fl oz	0	0	0
***Mountain Dew**	12 fl oz	180	0	0
***Mr. Pibb**	12 fl oz	140	0	0
Orange Soda (Store Brand):				
*Diet	12 fl oz	1	0	0
*Regular	12 fl oz	180	0	0
Pepsi-Cola:				
*Diet	12 fl oz	1	0	0
*Regular	12 fl oz	160	0	0
Pepsi-Free:				
*Diet	12 fl oz	1	0	0
*Regular	12 fl oz	160	0	0
***Quinine Water** (Store Brand)	12 fl oz	125	0	0
***Root Beer Ramblin'**	12 fl oz	180	0	0
Slice:				
*Diet	12 fl oz	1	0	0
*Regular	12 fl oz	150	0	0
Sprite:				
*Diet	12 fl oz	1	0	0
*Regular	12 fl oz	142	0	0

FOOD	MEASURE OR QUANTITY	CALORIES	FAT GRAMS	% FAT
*Tab	12 fl oz	1	0	0
Tonic Water (Store Brand):				
*Diet	12 fl oz	1	0	0
*Regular	12 fl oz	125	0	0

■ COCOA DRINKS
Fat Range = 0% to 30%
Average Fat = 12%

FOOD	MEASURE OR QUANTITY	CALORIES	FAT GRAMS	% FAT
*Alba Chocolate	1 envlp	62	0	0
Carnation:				
*Chocolate Rich	1 envlp	110	1	8
*Instant	1 envlp	110	1	8
*Instant and Marshmallow	1 envlp	110	1	8
*70 Calorie	1 envlp	70	0	0
*Sugar Free	1 envlp	50	0	0
*Nestle's Dry Chocolate Mix	2 oz	120	4	30
Hershey:				
*Dry Mix	2 oz	120	4	30
*Syrup	2 T	80	1	11
*Ovaltine Sugar Free	1 envlp	40	1	22
Swiss Miss:				
*Swiss Miss Chocolate	1 envlp	110	3	25
*Double Chocolate	1 envlp	110	3	25
*Lite	1 envlp	70	0	0
*and Marshmallows	1 envlp	110	3	25
*Sugar Free	1 envlp	50	0	0
*Sugar Free and Marshmallow	1 envlp	50	0	0

■ COFFEE
Fat Range = 0% to 77%
Average Fat = 37%

FOOD	MEASURE OR QUANTITY	CALORIES	FAT GRAMS	% FAT
Amaretto:				
(General Foods)	6 fl oz	51	2	35
Sugar Free (General Foods)	6 fl oz	36	3	75
*Cappuccino (General Foods)	6 fl oz	60	2	30
Francais:				
(General Foods)	6 fl oz	55	3	49
Sugar Free (General Foods)	6 fl oz	35	3	77
Irish Cream:				
(General Foods)	6 fl oz	55	3	49
Sugar Free (General Foods)	6 fl oz	32	2	56

FOOD	MEASURE OR QUANTITY	CALORIES	FAT GRAMS	% FAT
*Orange Cappuccino				
(General Foods)	6 fl oz	60	2	30
Regular:				
*Black	6 fl oz	4	0	0
*Black with 2 t Sugar	6 fl oz	34	0	0
*1 oz Skim Milk and 2 t Sugar	6 fl oz	44	0	0
*1 oz Whole Milk and 2 t Sugar	6 fl oz	55	1	16
Whole Milk, No Sugar	6 fl oz	22	1	41
Suisse Mocha:				
(General Foods)	6 fl oz	50	3	54
Sugar Free (General Foods)	6 fl oz	30	2	60
Vienna:				
*(General Foods)	6 fl oz	60	2	30
Sugar Free (General Foods)	6 fl oz	30	2	60

■ **FRUIT DRINKS**
READY TO DRINK—ALSO SEE JUICES
Fat Range = 0%
Average Fat = 0%

FOOD	MEASURE OR QUANTITY	CALORIES	FAT GRAMS	% FAT
Apple:				
*(Hi-C)	6 fl oz	90	0	0
*(Juice Works)	6 fl oz	100	0	0
*(Kool Aid)	8 fl oz	100	0	0
*(Ssipps)	8 fl oz	130	0	0
*(Wyler's)	8 fl oz	90	0	0
*Appleberry (Juice Works)	6 fl oz	100	0	0
*Apple Cranberry (Mott's)	10 fl oz	180	0	0
*Apple Raspberry (Mott's)	10 fl oz	150	0	0
*Apple Strawberry (Mott's)	10 fl oz	170	0	0
Cherry:				
*(Hi-C)	6 fl oz	90	0	0
*(Juice Works)	6 fl oz	100	0	0
*(Kool Aid)	8 fl oz	90	0	0
*Sugar Free (Kool Aid)	8 fl oz	4	0	0
*Citrus Cooler (Hi-C)	6 fl oz	90	0	0
Cranberry Apple:				
*Low Calorie (Ocean Spray)	6 fl oz	30	0	0
*(Ocean Spray)	6 fl oz	130	0	0
*Cranberry Apricot				
(Ocean Spray)	6 fl oz	110	0	0
*Cranberry Orange				
(Ocean Spray)	6 fl oz	100	0	0
*Fruit Juicy Red				
(Hawaiian Punch)	6 fl oz	90	0	0
*Fruit Punch (Mott's)	10 fl oz	170	0	0
*Fruit Punch (Ssipps)	9 fl oz	130	0	0
Grape:				
*Frozen (Welch's)	6 fl oz	90	0	0

FOOD	MEASURE OR QUANTITY	CALORIES	FAT GRAMS	% FAT
*(Hawaiian Punch)	6 fl oz	90	0	0
*(Juice Works)	6 fl oz	100	0	0
*(Kool Aid)	6 fl oz	90	0	0
*(Ssipps)	9 fl oz	130	0	0
*Sugar Free (Kool Aid)	6 fl oz	4	0	0
*(Tang)	6 fl oz	90	0	0
*(Welchaid)	6 fl oz	90	0	0
*(Welch's)	6 fl oz	110	0	0
*Grapefruit (Tang)	6 fl oz	90	0	0
*Island Fruit Cocktail				
(Hawaiian Punch)	6 fl oz	90	0	0
Lemon Lime:				
*(Country Time)	6 fl oz	70	0	0
*(Ssipps)	9 fl oz	85	0	0
Lemonade:				
*(Country Time)	6 fl oz	70	0	0
*(Crystal Light)	6 fl oz	4	0	0
*(Kool Aid)	6 fl oz	70	0	0
*(Minute Maid)	6 fl oz	75	0	0
*Mix (Wyler's)	6 fl oz	70	0	0
Lemonade, Pink:				
*(Country Time)	6 fl oz	70	0	0
*(Kool Aid)	6 fl oz	70	0	0
Lemonade, Sugar Free:				
*(Country Time)	6 fl oz	4	0	0
*(Kool Aid)	6 fl oz	4	0	0
*(Store Brand)	6 fl oz	4	0	0
*(Wyler's)	6 fl oz	4	0	0
*Limeade (Minute Maid)	6 fl oz	75	0	0
*Lite Fruit Juicy Red				
(Hawaiian Punch)	6 fl oz	60	0	0
*Mixed Berry (Ssipps)	9 fl oz	130	0	0
Orange:				
*(Crystal Light)	6 fl oz	4	0	0
*(Hawaiian Punch)	6 fl oz	100	0	0
*(Juice Works)	6 fl oz	90	0	0
*(Kool Aid)	6 fl oz	90	0	0
*(Ssipps)	9 fl oz	130	0	0
*(Tang)	6 fl oz	90	0	0
Punch:				
*Crystal Light	6 fl oz	4	0	0
*Hi-C	6 fl oz	100	0	0
*Kool Aid	6 fl oz	100	0	0
*(Wyler's)	6 fl oz	90	0	0
Punch, Sugar Free:				
*(Kool Aid)	6 fl oz	4	0	0
*(Wyler's)	6 fl oz	4	0	0
*Raspberry (Kool Aid)	6 fl oz	70	0	0
Strawberry:				
*(Hi-C)	6 fl oz	100	0	0
*(Juice Works)	6 fl oz	100	0	0
*(Kool Aid)	6 fl oz	90	0	0
*Sunshine Punch (Ssipps)	9 fl oz	130	0	0
*Tropical Fruit (Hawaiian Punch)	6 fl oz	90	0	0
*Very Berry (Hawaiian Punch)	6 fl oz	90	0	0

FOOD	MEASURE OR QUANTITY	CALORIES	FAT GRAMS	% FAT
*Wild Berry (Hi-C)	6 fl oz	90	0	0
Wild Cherry:				
*(Ssipps)	9 fl oz	130	0	0
*Sugar Free (Wyler's)	6 fl oz	4	0	0
*(Wyler's)	6 fl oz	70	0	0
*Wild Fruit (Hawaiian Punch)	6 fl oz	90	0	0
Wild Grape:				
*Sugar Free (Wyler's)	6 fl oz	4	0	0
*(Wyler's)	6 fl oz	90	0	0

■ **T E A**
Fat Range = 0% to 47%
Average Fat = 9%

FOOD	MEASURE OR QUANTITY	CALORIES	FAT GRAMS	% FAT
*Herbal	6 fl oz	1	0	0
Regular:				
*With Lemon	6 fl oz	1	0	0
*With 1 oz Skim Milk	6 fl oz	12	0	0
With 1 oz Whole Milk	6 fl oz	19	1	47
*With 2t Sugar and Lemon	6 fl oz	31	0	0
*With 2t Sugar and 1 oz Skim Milk	6 fl oz	41	0	0
*With 2t Sugar and 1 oz Whole Milk	6 fl oz	48	1	19

5. BREAKFAST FOODS

The cold cereals are listed without milk. The milk values should be used in addition to the value listed next to the cold cereal.

■ **M I L K**
Fat Range = 0% to 49%
Average Fat = 31%

FOOD	MEASURE OR QUANTITY	CALORIES	FAT GRAMS	% FAT
1% Fat	4 fl oz	53	2	34
2% Fat	4 fl oz	65	3	41

FOOD	MEASURE OR QUANTITY	CALORIES	FAT GRAMS	% FAT
*Skim	4 fl oz	45	0	0
Whole, Regular	4 fl oz	74	4	49

■ COLD CEREALS
1 OZ OF CEREAL IS EQUAL TO APPROX 1 CUP
Fat Range = 0% to 26%
Average Fat = 9%

FOOD	MEASURE OR QUANTITY	CALORIES	FAT GRAMS	% FAT
*All Bran (Kellogg's)	1 oz	70	1	13
*Almond Delight (Kellogg's)	1 oz	110	2	16
*AlphaBits (Post)	1 oz	110	1	8
*Apple Cinnamon Cheerios (General Mills)	1 oz	110	2	16
*Apple-Jacks (Kellogg's)	1 oz	110	0	0
*Apple Raisin Crisps (Kellogg's)	1 oz	120	0	0
*Batman (Ralston)	1 oz	110	1	8
*Body Buddies Fruit Flavor (General Mills)	1 oz	110	1	8
*Boo*Berry (General Mills)	1 oz	110	1	8
*Bran 100% (Nabisco)	1 oz	70	2	26
*Bran-Buds (Kellogg's)	1 oz	70	1	13
*Bran Chex (Ralston)	1 oz	90	1	10
Bran Flakes:				
*(Kellogg's)	1 oz	90	0	0
*40% (Post)	1 oz	90	0	0
*40% (Ralston)	1 oz	90	0	0
*Bran Muffin Crisps (General Mills)	1 oz	130	1	7
*Breakfast with Barbie (Ralston)	1 oz	110	1	8
C. W. Post Hearty Granola:				
*Regular (Post)	1 oz	130	4	28
*With Raisins (Post)	1 oz	120	4	30
*Cap'n Crunch (Quaker)	1 oz	120	3	22
*Cheerios (General Mills)	1 oz	110	2	16
*Choco Crunch (Quaker)	1 oz	116	2	16
*Cinnamon Toast Crunch (General Mills)	1 oz	120	3	22
*Circus Fun (General Mills)	1 oz	110	1	8
*Cocoa Krispies (Kellogg's)	1 oz	110	0	0
*Cocoa Pebbles (Post)	1 oz	110	1	8
*Cocoa Puffs (General Mills)	1 oz	110	1	8
*Cookie Crisp, Chocolate Flavor (Ralston)	1 oz	110	1	8
*Corn Bran (Quaker)	1 oz	110	1	8
*Corn Chex (Ralston)	1 oz	110	0	0
Corn Flakes:				
*Country (General Mills)	1 oz	110	0	0
*(Kellogg's)	1 oz	110	0	0
*(Ralston)	1 oz	110	0	0
*Post Toasties (Post)	1 oz	110	0	0

FOOD	MEASURE OR QUANTITY	CALORIES	FAT GRAMS	% FAT
*Corn Pops (Kellogg's)	1 oz	110	0	0
*Corn Total (General Mills)	1 oz	110	1	8
*Count Chocula (General Mills)	1 oz	110	1	8
Cracklin' Oat Bran (Kellogg's)	1 oz	110	4	33
*Crispix (Kellogg's)	1 oz	110	0	0
*Crispy Rice (Ralston)	1 oz	110	0	0
*Crunch Berries (Quaker)	1 oz	120	3	22
*Donkey Kong (Ralston)	1 oz	110	1	8
*Donkey Kong, Junior (Ralston)	1 oz	110	1	8
*Fiber One (General Mills)	1 oz	60	1	15
*Fortified Oat Flakes (Post)	1 oz	100	1	9
*Frankenberry (General Mills)	1 oz	110	1	8
*Froot Loops (Kellogg's)	1 oz	110	1	8
*Frosted Flakes (Kellogg's)	1 oz	110	0	0
*Frosted Mini-Wheats (Kellogg's)	4	110	0	0
*Fruit & Fibre, Apples & Cinnamon (Post)	1 oz	90	1	10
*Fruit Rings (Ralston)	1 oz	110	1	8
*Fruitful Bran (Kellogg's)	1 oz	115	0	0
*Golden Grahams (General Mills)	1 oz	110	1	8
*Grape-Nuts Flakes (Post)	1 oz	100	1	9
*Grape-Nuts (Post)	1 oz	110	0	0
*Halfsies (Quaker)	1 oz	112	1	8
*Heartwise (Kellogg's)	1 oz	90	1	10
Honey Bunches of Oats:				
*With Almonds (Post)	1 oz	120	3	22
*With Honey (Post)	1 oz	110	2	16
*Honey Nut Cheerios (General Mills)	1 oz	110	1	8
*Honey Nut Corn Flakes (Kellogg's)	1 oz	110	1	8
*Honey Nut Crunch Raisin Bran (Post)	1 oz	90	1	10
*Honey Smacks (Kellogg's)	1 oz	110	0	0
*Honeycomb (Post)	1 oz	110	1	8
*Just Right (Kellogg's)	1 oz	100	0	0
*Kabooms (General Mills)	1 oz	110	1	8
*Kix (General Mills)	1 oz	110	1	8
Life (Quaker):				
Cinnamon	1 oz	110	5	41
*Plain	1 oz	111	2	16
*Raisin	1 oz	105	2	17
*Lucky Charms (General Mills)	1 oz	110	1	8
*Marshmallow Krispies (Kellogg's)	1 oz	140	0	0
*Mueslix Bran (Kellogg's)	1 oz	130	2	14
*Muesli (Ralston)	1 oz	160	3	17
*Nut & Honey Crunch (Kellogg's)	1 oz	110	1	8
Nutri-Grain (Kellogg's):				
*Almond Raisin	1 oz	150	2	12
*Corn	1 oz	100	1	9
*Wheat	1 oz	100	0	0
*Nutrific (Kellogg's)	1 oz	120	2	15
*Oatbake (Kellogg's)	1 oz	110	3	25
*Oh's Apple Cinnamon, Honey Grahams	1 oz	120	2	15
*Pac-Man (General Mills)	1 oz	110	1	8

FOOD	MEASURE OR QUANTITY	CALORIES	FAT GRAMS	% FAT
*Peanut Butter Cereal (Quaker)	1 oz	130	4	28
*Product 19 (Kellogg's)	1 oz	110	0	0
*Pro Grain (Kellogg's)	1 oz	100	0	0
*Puffed Rice (Quaker)	1 oz	55	0	0
*Puffed Wheat (Quaker)	1 oz	54	0	0
Raisin Bran:				
*(Post)	1 oz	80	0	0
*(Kellogg's)	1 oz	120	1	8
*(Ralston)	1 oz	120	0	0
*Raisin Grape-Nuts (Post)	1 oz	100	0	0
*Raisin Nut Bran (General Mills)	1 oz	110	3	25
*Raisin Squares (Kellogg's)	1 oz	90	0	0
*Rice Chex (Ralston)	1 oz	110	0	0
*Rice Krispies (Kellogg's)	1 oz	110	0	0
*Rocky Road (General Mills)	1 oz	120	3	22
*S'Mores (General Mills)	1 oz	120	2	15
Shredded Wheat:				
*(Nabisco)	1 biscuit	90	1	10
*(Quaker)	2 biscuit	104	1	9
*Spoon Size (Nabisco)	1 oz	110	0	0
*Smurf-Berry Crunch (Post)	1 oz	110	1	8
*Special K (Kellogg's)	1 oz	110	0	0
*Strawberry Squares (Kellogg's)	1 oz	90	0	0
*Sugar Frosted Flakes (Ralston)	1 oz	110	1	8
*Sugar Frosted Rice (Ralston)	1 oz	110	0	0
*Super Golden Crisps (Post)	1 oz	110	0	0
*Tasteeos (Ralston)	1 oz	110	0	0
*Teddy Grahams	1 oz	120	3	22
*Teenage Mutant Ninja Turtles				
(Ralston)	1 oz	110	0	0
*Toasted Wheat & Raisins				
(Nabisco)	1 oz	100	1	9
*Total (General Mills)	1 oz	110	1	8
*Trix (General Mills)	1 oz	110	1	8
*Tropical Fruit (Post)	1 oz	110	1	8
*Wheat Chex (Ralston)	1 oz	100	0	0
Wheat Germ:				
*Honey Toasted (Kretschmer)	3 T	110	3	25
*Toasted (Kretschmer)	3 T	100	3	27
*Wheat & Raisin Chex (Ralston)	1 oz	130	0	0
*Wheaties (General Mills)	1 oz	110	1	8

■ CROISSANTS
Fat Range = 38% to 49%
Average Fat = 42%

FOOD	MEASURE OR QUANTITY	CALORIES	FAT GRAMS	% FAT
Almond (Pepperidge Farm)	1	210	11	47
Butter:				
Original (Sara Lee)	1	170	9	47
Petite (Sara Lee)	1	120	6	45

FOOD	MEASURE OR QUANTITY	CALORIES	FAT GRAMS	% FAT
Cheese (Sara Lee)	1	170	9	48
Chocolate (Pepperidge Farm)	1	260	16	55
Raisin (Pepperidge Farm)	1	210	10	43
Sandwich:				
Chicken and Broccoli (Sara Lee)	1	340	17	45
Ham and Swiss Cheese (Sara Lee)	1	340	18	48
Turkey, Bacon and Cheese (Sara Lee)	1	370	20	49

■ HOT CEREALS
Fat Range = 0% to 26%
Average Fat = 10%

FOOD	MEASURE OR QUANTITY	CALORIES	FAT GRAMS	% FAT
*Cream of Rice (Nabisco)	1 oz	110	1	8
*Cream of Wheat, Instant (Nabisco)	1 oz	100	0	0
*Cream of Wheat, Regular (Nabisco)	¾ cup	110	1	8
Cream of Wheat, Mix n Eat:				
*Apple Cinnamon (Nabisco)	1-¼ oz	130	0	0
*Brown Sugar (Nabisco)	1-¼ oz	130	0	0
*Maple Sugar (Nabisco)	1-¼ oz	130	0	0
*Original (Nabisco)	1-¼ oz	100	0	0
*Peach (Nabisco)	1-¼ oz	140	2	13
*Farina (Pillsbury)	2/3 cup	80	1	11
*Maltex Old Fashioned (Uhliman)	½ cup	90	1	10
Maypo:				
*30 Second (Uhliman)	½ cup	110	1	8
*Vermont Style (Uhliman)	½ cup	90	0	0
Oat Bran, Hearty:				
*Honey Flavored (Nabisco)	1 pkg	110	0	0
*Regular (Nabisco)	1 pkg	80	2	22
Oatmeal, Instant:				
*Apple and Cinnamon (Quaker)	¾ cup	135	2	13
*Apple Raisin Walnut (Quaker)	¾ cup	130	3	21
*Bran and Raisins (Quaker)	¾ cup	155	2	12
*Cinnamon and Spice (Quaker)	¾ cup	160	2	11
*Honey and Graham (Quaker)	¾ cup	136	2	13
*Maple and Brown Sugar (Quaker)	¾ cup	163	2	11
*Peaches and Cream (Quaker)	¾ cup	130	2	14
*Raisin and Dates (Quaker)	¾ cup	150	4	24
*Raisin and Spice (Quaker)	¾ cup	150	2	12
*Regular (Quaker)	¾ cup	105	2	17
*Strawberries (Quaker)	¾ cup	136	2	13
Oatmeal, Swirlers:				
*Apple Cinnamon (General Mills)	1 pkg	160	2	11
*Cherry (General Mills)	1 pkg	150	2	12

FOOD	MEASURE OR QUANTITY	CALORIES	FAT GRAMS	% FAT
*Chocolate (General Mills)	1 pkg	170	2	11
*Strawberry (General Mills)	1 pkg	150	2	12
Oatmeal, Total:				
*Apple Cinnamon				
(General Mills)	1 pkg	130	2	14
*Mixed Nut (General Mills)	1 pkg	140	4	26
*Quick (General Mills)	1 pkg	90	2	20
*Ralston, Regular				
(Ralston Purina)	4 fl oz	90	0	0
*Wheat Hearts (General Mills)	¾ cup	110	1	8
*Wheatena (Uhliman)	½ cup	80	0	0

■ **PANCAKES**

Fat Range = 13% to 42%
Average Fat = 21%
Pancakes are 4″ diameter

FOOD	MEASURE OR QUANTITY	CALORIES	FAT GRAMS	% FAT
*Batter, Froz. (Aunt Jemina)	3	210	3	13
Blueberry:				
*Complete (Aunt Jemima)	3	230	4	16
*Frozen (Aunt Jemima)	3	210	3	13
(Hungry Jack)	3	320	15	42
*Pancake Express				
(Aunt Jemima)	3	230	4	16
*Buckwheat, Homemade	3	160	3	17
Buttermilk:				
(Betty Crocker)	3	280	10	32
*Frozen (Aunt Jemima)	3	250	4	14
*Homemade	3	160	3	17
(Hungry Jack)	3	240	11	41
*Lite (Aunt Jemima)	3	140	3	19
*Lite Express (Aunt Jemima)	3	130	2	14
Original:				
*(Aunt Jemima)	3	260	4	14
*Complete (Aunt Jemima)	3	240	3	11
*Pancake Express				
(Aunt Jemima)	3	240	3	11
*Pancakes with Blueberry				
Sauce, Frozen (Swanson)	7 oz pkg	400	9	20
Pancakes with Sausage, Frozen				
(Swanson)	6 oz pkg	460	22	43
*Pancakes with Strawberry,				
Frozen (Swanson)	7 oz pkg	430	8	17
Plain:				
*Extra Lights (Hungry Jack)	3	210	7	30
*(Golden Blend)	3	240	5	19
*Homemade	3	150	3	18
*Packets (Hungry Jack)	3	180	3	15

■ TOASTER CAKES
Fat Range = 19% to 34%
Average Fat = 24%

FOOD	MEASURE OR QUANTITY	CALORIES	FAT GRAMS	% FAT
*All Flavors, Toastettes				
(Nabisco)	1	200	5	23
*Apple, Dutch, Pop-Tarts				
(Kellogg's)	1	210	6	26
*Blueberry:				
*Frosted, Pop-Tarts (Kellogg's)	1	200	5	23
*Pop-Tarts (Kellogg's)	1	210	5	21
Toaster Strudel (Pillsbury)	1	190	8	38
*Brown Sugar, Pop-Tarts				
(Kellogg's)	1	200	5	23
*Cherry, Pop-Tarts (Kellogg's)	1	210	5	21
*Chocolate Fudge, Pop-Tarts				
(Kellogg's)	1	200	4	18
*Chocolate Vanilla, Pop-Tarts				
(Kellogg's)	1	220	6	25
Cinnamon, Toaster Strudel				
(Pillsbury)	1	190	8	38
*Grape, Concord, Pop-Tarts				
(Kellogg's)	1	210	6	27
Raspberry:				
*Pop-Tarts (Kellogg's)	1	210	6	26
Toaster Strudel (Pillsbury)	1	190	8	38
Strawberry:				
*Pop-Tarts (Kellogg's)	1	210	6	26
Toaster Strudel (Pillsbury)	1	190	8	38

■ WAFFLES AND FRENCH TOAST
Fat Range = 21% to 47%
Average Fat = 33%

FOOD	MEASURE OR QUANTITY	CALORIES	FAT GRAMS	% FAT
*Apple and Cinnamon				
(Aunt Jemina)	2	170	4	21
Blueberry:				
*(Aunt Jemina)	2	170	4	21
(Eggo)	1	130	5	35
Bran (Eggo)	1	170	8	42
Bran, Blueberries (Eggo)	1	130	5	35
Bran, Strawberries (Eggo)	1	120	5	38
Buttermilk:				
*(Aunt Jemima)	2	175	4	21
(Eggo)	1	120	5	38
French Toast:				
*(Aunt Jemima)	2	170	5	26

FOOD	MEASURE OR QUANTITY	CALORIES	FAT GRAMS	% FAT
*Cinnamon Swirl				
(Aunt Jemima)	2	210	7	30
(Downyflake)	2	270	14	47
(Homemade)	2	200	7	32
*Raisin (Aunt Jemima)	2	190	5	24
Nutrigrain (Eggo)	1	130	5	35
Plain:				
(Eggo)	1	120	5	38
(Homemade)	7″ Dia	200	8	36
(Roman Meal)	1	140	7	45

6. CONDIMENTS

■ CONDIMENTS
ADDITIONAL REFERENCES IN SAUCES AND SALAD DRESSINGS
Fat Range = 0% to 97%
Average Fat = 15%

FOOD	MEASURE OR QUANTITY	CALORIES	FAT GRAMS	% FAT
*Allspice, Ground	1 t	5	0	0
*Anise Seed	1 t	7	0	0
Bacon Bits:				
Bac Os (General Mills)	1 T	30	2	30
(Durkee)	1 T	44	2	41
(Hormel)	1 T	30	2	60
Bacon Chips (McCormick)	1 T	28	1	32
*Bay Leaf	1 t	2	0	0
*Beets, Dilled (Catelli)	3 pieces	20	0	0
*Butter Salt	1 T	0	0	0
*Cardamom Ground	1 t	6	0	0
*Catsup (Del Monte)	2 fl oz	60	0	0
*Celery Seed	1 t	8	0	0
*Cinnamon, Ground	1 t	6	0	0
*Cumin Seed	1 t	8	0	0
*Curry Powder	1 T	0	0	0
*Curry Powder	1 t	0	0	0
*Fennel Seed	1 t	7	0	0
*Garlic Salt	1 T	0	0	0
Gherkins:				
*Large	1	50	0	0
*Medium	1	20	0	0

FOOD	MEASURE OR QUANTITY	CALORIES	FAT GRAMS	% FAT
Sweet:				
*(Catelli)	3	25	0	0
*(Heinz)	1 oz	35	0	0
*Ginger	1 t	5	0	0
*Hamburger Relish (Heinz)	1 oz	30	0	0
Horseradish:				
*(Gold's)	1 T	4	0	0
*(Kraft)	1 T	4	0	0
Horseradish Sauce (Kraft)	1 T	50	5	90
*Hot Dog Relish (Heinz)	1 oz	35	0	0
*India Relish (Heinz)	1 oz	35	0	0
*Jalapeño Peppers (Vlassic)	1 oz	8	0	0
*Lemon Pepper	1 T	0	0	0
*Marjoram	1 t	2	0	0
*Meat Tenderizer (McCormick)	1 t	2	0	0
Mustard, Brown 'n Spicy				
(R.T. French)	1 T	10	1	90
*Mustard, Dijon (R.T. French)	1 T	8	0	0
*Mustard Seed	1 t	15	0	0
*Nutmeg	1 t	12	0	0
Olives:				
Colossal	10	95	10	95
Giant	10	65	7	97
Greek Style	10	65	7	97
*Onion Salt	1 T	0	0	0
*Oregano	1 t	5	0	0
*Parsley	1 t	1	0	0
*Pepper	1 T	0	0	0
Pickles, Dill				
*Featherweight	1	4	0	0
*Kosher (Featherweight)	1	10	0	0
*Kosher (Vlassic)	1 oz	4	0	0
*Spears (Vlassic)	1 oz	4	0	0
*Pickles, Sour	1	14	0	0
*Pickles, Sweet Mixed (Heinz)	1 oz	40	0	0
*Poppy Seed	1 t	15	0	0
*Poultry Seasoning	1 T	0	0	0
*Saffron	1 t	2	0	0
*Sage	1 t	2	0	0
*Salt Substitute	1 T	0	0	0
Sauerkraut:				
*(Vlassic)	1 oz	4	0	0
*(Vlassic)	1 cup	50	0	0
*Seafood Cocktail, Tomato				
(Del Monte)	2 fl oz	70	0	0
*Seasoned Salt	1 T	0	0	0
*Soy Sauce (Store Brand)	1 T	15	0	0
*Thyme	1 t	5	0	0
*Turmeric	1 t	8	0	0
*Vinegar (Store Brand)	1 T	2	0	0

■ CROUTONS
Fat Range = 30% to 51%
Average Fat = 41%

FOOD	MEASURE OR QUANTITY	CALORIES	FAT GRAMS	% FAT
Bacon and Cheese				
(Pepperidge Farm)	½ oz	70	3	39
Blue Cheese (Pepperidge Farm)	½ oz	70	4	51
Caesar (Brownsberry)	½ oz	70	3	39
Cheddar (Brownberry)	½ oz	65	3	42
***Cheddar and Romano**				
(Pepperidge Farm)	½ oz	60	2	30
Cheese and Garlic				
(Pepperidge Farm)	½ oz	70	3	39
Dijon Mustard				
(Pepperidge Farm)	½ oz	70	4	51
Onion and Garlic				
(Pepperidge Farm)	½ oz	70	3	39
Ranch Style (Brownberry)	½ oz	65	3	42
Sour Cream and Chive				
(Pepperidge Farm)	½ oz	70	3	39
Toasted-Brownberry	½ oz	65	3	42

■ SALAD DRESSINGS
Fat Range = 0% to 100%
Average Fat = 65%

FOOD	MEASURE OR QUANTITY	CALORIES	FAT GRAMS	% FAT
Bacon and Buttermilk (Kraft)	1 T	80	8	90
Bacon, Creamy:				
Reduced (Kraft)	1 T	30	2	60
(Seven Seas)	1 T	60	6	90
Bacon and Tomato, Reduced				
(Kraft)	1 T	30	2	60
Blue Cheese:				
*(Estee)	1 T	8	0	0
(Hain)	1 T	70	7	90
(Marie's Lite)	1 T	40	4	90
(Walden Farms)	1 T	27	2	67
(Weight Watchers)	1 T	10	1	90
(Wish-Bone Lite)	1 T	40	3	68
Blue Cheese Chunky:				
(Kraft)	1 T	70	6	77
(Kraft Reduced)	1 T	30	2	60
(Wish-Bone)	1 T	70	7	90
Blue Cheese and Herbs Mix				
(Good Seasons)	1 T	73	8	99
Buttermilk:				
*Creamy (Estee)	1 T	6	0	0
Creamy, Reduced (Kraft)	1 T	30	3	90

FOOD	MEASURE OR QUANTITY	CALORIES	FAT GRAMS	% FAT
(Seven Seas)	1 T	40	4	90
(Wish-Bone)	1 T	50	5	90
Ceasar (Wish-Bone)	1 T	70	7	90
Cheddar and Bacon				
(Wish-Bone)	1 T	70	7	90
Cheese Avocado (Hain)	1 T	70	7	90
Cheese Italian (Good Seasons)	1 T	73	8	99
Cucumber (Hain)	1 T	80	8	90
Cucumber, Creamy:				
*(Herb Magic)	1 T	8	0	0
(Kraft)	1 T	73	8	99
(Kraft Reduced)	1 T	30	3	90
(Wish-Bone)	1 T	80	8	90
(Wish-Bone Lite)	1 T	40	4	90
***Dijon, Creamy** (Estee)	1 T	8	0	0
Dijon French Vinaigrette				
(Wish-Bone)	1 T	61	6	89
French:				
Capri (Seven Seas)	1 T	70	6	77
Deluxe (Wish-Bone)	1 T	50	5	90
(Homemade)	1 T	100	10	90
(Kraft)	1 T	60	6	90
Lite (Store Brand)	1 T	25	1	36
Lite (Wish-Bone)	1 T	30	2	60
Reduced (Kraft)	1 T	25	2	72
Sweet and Spicy (Wish-Bone)	1 T	70	6	77
(Walden Farms)	1 T	33	2	55
***French, Creamy** (Estee)	1 T	4	0	0
French, Garlic (Wish-Bone)	1 T	60	6	90
French, Herbal (Wish-Bone)	1 T	60	6	90
Garden Herb (Hidden Valley Ranch)	1 T	70	7	90
Garlic, Creamy (Wish-Bone)	1 T	80	8	90
Garlic and Herb (Good Seasons)	1 T	84	9	96
Green Goddess (Seven Seas)	1 T	65	7	97
Herbs and Spices (Seven Seas)	1 T	60	6	90
Italian:				
(Good Seasons)	1 T	73	8	99
*(Herb Magic)	1 T	4	0	0
*(Homemade)	1 T	70	7	90
*(Kraft)	1 T	4	0	0
*Low Calorie (Good Seasons)	1 T	8	0	0
*(Richard Simmons)	1 spray	1	0	0
(Seven Seas)	1 T	70	7	90
*(Walden Farms)	1 T	9	0	0
*(Weight Watchers)	1 T	2	0	0
(Wish-Bone)	1 T	70	7	90
Italian, Creamy:				
*(Estee)	1 T	4	0	0
(Hain)	1 T	80	8	90
Lite (Wish-Bone)	1 T	30	3	90
Low Fat (Walden Farms)	1 T	35	3	77
(Seven Seas)	1 T	70	7	90
(Weight Watchers)	1 T	50	5	90
Italian Garlic (Marie's Lite)	1 T	36	3	75
Italian, Herbal (Wish-Bone)	1 T	70	7	90

FOOD	MEASURE OR QUANTITY	CALORIES	FAT GRAMS	% FAT
Italian, Lite:				
(Good Seasons)	1 T	30	3	90
*(Kraft Reduced)	1 T	6	0	0
Store Brand	1 T	20	2	90
(Wish-Bone)	1 T	30	3	90
Italian, Mild (Seven Seas)	1 T	70	7	90
***Italian, No Oil** (Good Seasons)	1 T	7	0	0
Italian Ranch (Marie's Lite)	1 T	36	3	75
Italian, Zesty:				
*(Estee)	1 T	4	0	0
(Good Seasons)	1 T	73	8	99
Lite (Good Seasons)	1 T	31	3	87
Mayonnaise Dressing				
(Homemade)	1 T	60	5	75
Oil (All Types)	1 T	126	14	100
Oil and Vinegar (Kraft)	1 T	70	7	90
Onion and Chives:				
(Kraft)	1 T	70	7	90
(Wish-Bone Lite)	1 T	40	3	68
Parmesan, Viva (Seven Seas)	1 T	60	6	90
Ranch:				
(Marie's Lite)	1 T	40	3	68
Original (Hidden Valley)	1 T	70	7	90
(Walden Farms)	1 T	35	2	51
Rancher's Choice (Kraft)	1 T	80	8	90
***Roma, Spray**				
(Richard Simmons)	1 spray	1	0	0
Romano (Hain)	1 T	73	8	99
Romano and Parmesan				
(Wish-Bone)	1 T	90	9	90
Russian:				
(Hain)	1 T	60	5	75
(Homemade)	1 T	80	8	90
(Kraft)	1 T	60	5	75
Lite (Store Brand)	1 T	25	1	36
*Reduced Calorie (Kraft)	1 T	18	0	0
(Wish-Bone)	1 T	45	2	40
Russian, Creamy				
(Seven Seas)	1 T	80	8	90
Sour Cream and Bacon				
(Wish-Bone)	1 T	70	7	90
Sour Cream and Dill				
(Marie's Lite)	1 T	50	4	72
***Sweet 'n Sour** (Herb Magic)	1 T	18	0	0
Thousand Island:				
*(Estee)	1 T	6	0	0
(Hain)	1 T	50	5	90
(Homemade)	1 T	60	6	90
(Seven Seas)	1 T	50	5	90
(Walden Farms)	1 T	24	2	75
(Weight Watchers)	1 T	12	1	75
(Wish-Bone)	1 T	60	6	90
Thousand Island Bacon:				
(Kraft)	1 T	60	6	90
(Wish-Bone)	1 T	60	6	90

FOOD	MEASURE OR QUANTITY	CALORIES	FAT GRAMS	% FAT
Thousand Island, Lite:				
(Kraft)	1 T	30	2	60
(Marie's)	1 T	40	3	68
(Store Brand)	1 T	25	1	36
(Wish-Bone)	1 T	25	2	72
***Vinaigrette** (Herb Magic)	1 T	6	0	0
***Vinegar, Balsamic**	1 T	2	0	0
***Vinegar** (Heinz)	1 T	2	0	0
***Vinegar, White** (Heinz)	1 T	2	0	0
Vinegar and Oil (Homemade)	1 T	73	8	99
***Zesty Tomato** (Herb Magic)	1 T	14	0	0

7. DAIRY PRODUCTS

■ CHEESE

Fat Range = 7% to 88%
Average Fat = 63%

FOOD	MEASURE OR QUANTITY	CALORIES	FAT GRAMS	% FAT
American, Processed	1 oz	105	9	77
Blue	1 oz	100	8	72
Blue, Crumbled	1 cup	479	39	73
Brick	1 oz	104	8	69
Brie	1 oz	96	8	75
Camembert	1 oz	113	9	72
Caraway	1 oz	104	8	69
Cheddar	1 oz	109	9	74
Cheddar, Cubed	1" cube	74	6	73
Cheddar, Shredded	1 cup	440	36	74
Cheese Spread	1 oz	82	6	66
Chesire	1 oz	113	9	72
Colby	1 oz	113	9	72
Cottage Cheese:				
*1% Fat	1 cup	154	2	12
*2% Fat	1 cup	192	4	19
4%, Large Curd	1 cup	206	10	44
4%, Small Curd	1 cup	209	9	39
*Uncreamed	1 cup	121	1	7
*Fruit	1 cup	280	8	26
Cream Cheese	1 oz	102	10	88
Edam	1 oz	100	8	72

FOOD	MEASURE OR QUANTITY	CALORIES	FAT GRAMS	% FAT
Feta	1 oz	74	6	73
Fontina	1 oz	109	9	74
Gjetost	1 oz	132	8	55
Gouda	1 oz	113	9	72
Gruyère	1 oz	113	9	72
Limburger	1 oz	96	8	75
Monterey Jack	1 oz	109	9	74
Mozzarella:				
Skim Milk	1 oz	77	5	58
Whole Milk	1 lb.	1300	100	69
Whole Milk	1 oz	82	6	66
Muenster	1 oz	109	9	74
Neufchâtel	1 oz	79	7	80
Parmesan, Grated	1 cup	454	30	59
Pimento, Proccesed	1 oz	105	9	77
Port-Du-Salut	1 oz	100	8	72
Provolone	1 oz	104	8	69
Ricotta:				
Skim Milk	1 cup	331	19	52
Whole Milk	1 cup	428	32	67
Romano	1 oz	112	8	64
Roquefort	1 oz	109	9	74
Swiss	1 oz	108	8	67
Swiss, Process	1 oz	95	7	66
Tilsit	1 oz	95	7	66
*Whey, Sweet	1 cup	69	1	13

■ CHEESE, PROCESSED
Fat Range = 0% to 90%
Average Fat = 65%

FOOD	MEASURE OR QUANTITY	CALORIES	FAT GRAMS	% FAT
American:				
(Borden's)	1 sl	110	9	74
(Kraft)	1 oz	90	7	70
(Kraft)	1 sl	110	9	74
Lite-Line (Kraft)	1 sl	110	9	74
(Lite 'n Lively)	1 sl	70	4	51
American, Sharp:				
(Kraft)	1 oz	110	9	74
(Kraft)	1 sl	110	9	74
Babybel (Bel Paese)	1 oz	91	7	69
Borden's Lite:				
American	1 oz	50	2	36
Cheddar	1 oz	80	5	56
Mozzarella	1 oz	50	2	36
Swiss	1 oz	50	2	36
Brick (Kraft)	1 oz	110	9	74
Caraway (Kraft)	1 oz	100	8	72
Cheddar, Imitation (Kraft)	1 oz	110	9	74

FOOD	MEASURE OR QUANTITY	CALORIES	FAT GRAMS	% FAT
Cheddar, Lite (Dorman's)	1 oz	90	7	70
Cheddar (Lite 'n Lively)	1 sl	70	4	51
Cheddar, Mild (Kraft)	1 oz	110	9	74
Cheddar, Port Wine				
(Cracker Barrel)	1 T	90	6	60
(Kraft)	1 oz	110	9	74
Cheddar, Sharp:				
(Wispread)	1 oz	100	7	63
Cheddar (Weight Watchers)	1 oz	80	5	56
Cheez Whiz:				
Mexican	1 oz	80	6	68
Pimento	1 oz	80	6	68
Regular	1 oz	80	6	68
Colby (Kraft)	1 oz	110	9	74
Cottage 4% (Borden's)	4 oz	120	5	38
*Cottage, Lofat (Lite Line)	4 oz	90	2	20
Cream Cheese, Philadelphia Brand (Kraft):				
Lite	1 oz	60	5	75
Plain	1 T	100	10	90
With Chives	1 T	100	10	90
With Pimento	1 T	100	10	90
Cream Cheese, Whipped, Philadelphia Brand (Kraft):				
Plain	1 T	100	10	90
With Bacon	1 T	100	10	90
With Onion	1 T	100	10	90
With Salmon	1 T	100	9	81
Edam (Kraft)	1 oz	100	8	72
Fior Di Latte (Polly-O)	1 oz	80	6	68
*Hoop (Friendship)	4 oz	120	0	0
Jalapeno Spread (Kraft)	1 oz	80	6	68
Laughing Cow	1	13	1	69
Mini Bonbel	1 oz	75	6	72
Monterey Jack (Kraft)	1 oz	110	9	74
Mozzarella:				
Sandwich (Polly-O)	1 oz	90	6	60
Skim (Polly-O)	1 oz	80	6	68
Smoked (Polly-O)	1 oz	80	5	56
Whole Milk (Polly-O)	1 oz	90	6	60
Muenster—Kraft	1 oz	100	8	72
Neufchatel (Kraft)	1 oz	80	7	79
Parmesan (Kraft)	1 T	130	9	62
Port Wine:				
(Weight Watchers)	2 T	70	4	51
Cheese, (Wispread)	1 oz	100	7	63
Provolone (Kraft)	1 oz	90	7	70
Ricotta, Skim (Polly-O)	2 oz	90	6	60
Ricotta, Whole Milk (Polly-O)	2 oz	100	7	63
Romano (Kraft)	1 oz	130	9	62
Sharp Cheddar (Weight Watcher's)	2 T	70	4	51
Squeez-A-Snack:				
Bacon	1 oz	90	7	70

FOOD	MEASURE OR QUANTITY	CALORIES	FAT GRAMS	% FAT
Garlic	1 oz	90	7	70
Hickory	1 oz	80	7	79
Sharp	1 oz	80	7	79
String Cheese (Polly-O)	1	90	6	60
Super Sharp (Hoffman)	1 oz	110	8	65
Swiss 'n Cheddar, Smoky (Hoffman)	1 oz	110	8	65
Swiss:				
(Kraft)	1 oz	100	8	72
(Lite Line)	1 oz	50	2	36
(Lite 'n Lively)	1 sl	70	4	51
Rye Cheese Food (Hoffman)	1 oz	90	7	70
Velveeta:				
Pimento Spread	1 oz	80	6	68
Slices	1 sl	90	6	60
Spread	1 oz	80	6	68

■ CHOCOLATE MILK

Fat Range = 5% to 35%

Average Fat = 22%

FOOD	MEASURE OR QUANTITY	CALORIES	FAT GRAMS	% FAT
Prepared with:				
*8 Ounces of 1% Milk	1	180	4	20
*8 Ounces of Skim Milk	1	170	1	5
*8 Ounces of 2% Milk	1	200	6	27
8 Ounces of Whole Milk	1	230	9	35

■ MILK AND CREAM

Fat Range = 0% to 88%

Average Fat = 44%

FOOD	MEASURE OR QUANTITY	CALORIES	FAT GRAMS	% FAT
Buttermilk:				
*Powdered	1 cup	303	7	21
*Regular	1 cup	98	2	18
Chocolate:				
*1% Fat	1 cup	163	3	17
Regular	1 cup	208	8	35
*2% Fat	1 cup	181	5	25
Chocolate Milkshake	1 cup	368	8	20
Condensed, Whole	1 cup	339	19	50
Condensed, Whole, Sweet	1 cup	1003	27	24

FOOD	MEASURE OR QUANTITY	CALORIES	FAT GRAMS	% FAT
Cream, Imitation:				
(Frozen)	1 cup	243	19	70
(Powdered)	1 cup	525	33	57
Cream, Light	1 cup	474	46	87
Cream, Whipped:				
Imitation	1 cup	192	16	75
Pressurized Can	1 cup	153	13	76
Cream, Whipping:				
Light	1 cup	705	73	93
Regular	1 cup	840	88	94
Eggnog	1 cup	347	19	49
Goat	1 cup	170	10	53
Half and Half	1 cup	320	28	79
Half and Half	1 T	22	2	82
Sour Cream:				
Non-fat	1 cup	427	39	82
Regular	1 cup	500	48	86
Soy	1 cup	89	5	51
Strawberry	1 cup	200	8	36
2% Fat	1 cup	125	5	36
***Whey, Sweet**	1 cup	69	107	28
Skim:				
*Evaporated	1 cup	201	1	4
*Evaporated	1 pkg	325	1	3
*Powdered	1 cup	240	0	0
*Regular	1 cup	89	1	10

■ **YOGURT**
 Fat Range = 0% to 39%
 Average Fat = 14%

FOOD	MEASURE OR QUANTITY	CALORIES	FAT GRAMS	% FAT
***Apple** (*Yoplait*)	6 oz	190	3	14
***Apple Cinnamon** (*Yoplait*)	6 oz	240	5	19
***Dutch Apple** (Dannon)	1 cup	240	3	11
Banana Strawberry:				
*(Colombo)	6 oz	180	1	5
*(Dannon Light)	1	100	0	0
Bavarian Chocolate (Colombo)	5 oz	270	11	37
***Berries** (*Yoplait*)	6 oz	230	5	20
Cherry:				
*(Dannon)	1 cup	260	3	10
*(La Yogurt)	1 cup	200	0	0
***Cherry, Black** (Light 'n Lively)	6 oz	180	2	10
Blueberry:				
*(Breyers)	1 cup	260	6	21
*(Colombo)	1 cup	160	1	6
*(Dannon Light)	1	100	0	0
*(La Yogurt)	1 cup	200	1	4
*(Light 'n Lively)	6 oz	180	2	10

FOOD	MEASURE OR QUANTITY	CALORIES	FAT GRAMS	% FAT
*Ultimate 90 (Weight Watchers)	1	90	0	0
*(Yoplait 150)	6 oz	150	0	0
*Cherries Jubilee, Ultimate 90				
(Weight Watchers)	1	90	0	0
Cherry Vanilla:				
*(Borden's)	1 cup	270	2	7
*(La Yogurt)	6 oz	190	4	19
*(Lite 'n Lively)	1 cup	240	2	8
Citrus Fruits:				
*(Yoplait)	6 oz	250	5	18
Coffee:				
*(Dannon)	1 cup	200	4	18
*(Yoplait)	6 oz	180	4	20
Fruit:				
*Low Fat (Store Brand)	4 oz	120	2	15
*Low Fat (Store Brand)	1 cup	240	4	15
*(Yes)	6 oz	190	4	19
*(Yoplait)	6 oz	190	4	19
*Fruit, Exotic (Dannon)	1 cup	240	3	11
*Fruit, Orchard (Yoplait)	6 oz	240	5	19
*Key Lime (La Yogurt)	6 oz	190	4	19
Lemon:				
*(Borden's)	1 cup	220	2	8
*Dannon	1 cup	200	4	18
*Ultimate 90 (Weight Watchers)	1	90	0	0
Mixed Berries:				
*(Breyers)	1 cup	270	5	17
*(Dannon)	1 cup	240	3	11
*(La Yogurt)	6 oz	190	4	19
*Mixed Berries & Nuts (Dannon)	1 cup	260	3	10
Peach:				
*(Breyers)	6 oz	270	5	17
*(Colombo)	1 cup	190	1	5
*(Dannon)	1 cup	260	2	7
*(Dannon Light)	1	100	0	0
*(Lite Line)	1 cup	230	2	8
*(Light 'n Lively)	6 oz	180	2	10
*Ultimate 90				
(Weight Watchers)	1	90	0	0
*(Yoplait 150)	6 oz	150	0	0
Pina Colada:				
*(Dannon)	1 cup	240	3	11
*(Yoplait)	4 oz	120	2	15
Pineapple:				
*(Borden's)	1 cup	260	2	7
*(Breyers)	1 cup	270	5	17
*(Light 'n Lively)	6 oz	180	2	10
Plain:				
(Breyers)	1 cup	190	8	38
*(Dannon)	1 cup	150	4	24
(La Yogurt)	6 oz	140	6	39
*(Lite Line)	1 cup	180	4	20
(Store Brand)	4 oz	70	3	39
(Store Brand)	1 cup	140	6	39
(Yoplait)	6 oz	130	5	35

FOOD	MEASURE OR QUANTITY	CALORIES	FAT GRAMS	% FAT
Plain, Low Fat:				
*(Store Brand)	4 oz	60	2	30
*(Store Brand)	1 cup	130	4	28
Plain with Honey (*Yoplait*)	6 oz	130	5	35
***Raspberry** (*Yoplait 150*)	6 oz	150	0	0
Red Raspberry:				
*(Breyers)	1 cup	260	6	21
*(Lite 'n Lively)	6 oz	170	2	11
Strawberry:				
*(Borden's)	1 cup	230	2	8
*(Breyers)	1 cup	270	5	17
*(Dannon)	1 cup	260	3	10
*(La Yogurt)	6 oz	190	4	19
*(La Yogurt 2)	1 cup	200	0	0
*Ultimate 90 (Weight Watchers)	1	90	0	0
Strawberry Banana:				
*(La Yogurt)	1 cup	200	0	0
*(La Yogurt)	6 oz	190	4	19
*(Light 'n Lively)	6 oz	200	2	9
*Ultimate 90 (Weight Watchers)	1	90	0	0
***Strawberry, Fruit in Cup** (La Yogurt)	6 oz	190	4	19
***Strawberry, Low Fat** (Colombo)	1 cup	190	0	0
***TCBY** (All Flavors)	6 oz	180	4	20
Tropical Fruit:				
*Ultimate 90 (Weight Watchers)	1	90	0	0
*(*Yoplait*)	6 oz	250	5	18
Vanilla:				
*(Dannon)	1 cup	200	4	18
*(*Yoplait*)	6 oz	180	4	20
***Vanilla Bean** (Breyers)	1 cup	230	7	27

8. DESSERTS AND PUDDINGS

■ CAKE FROSTINGS
1/12 OF PACKAGE OR 1 SLICE OF CAKE
Fat Range = 0% to 54%
Average Fat = 36%

FOOD	MEASURE OR QUANTITY	CALORIES	FAT GRAMS	% FAT
All Flavors, Creamy Deluxe (General Foods)	1/12	160	7	39

FOOD	MEASURE OR QUANTITY	CALORIES	FAT GRAMS	% FAT
Caramel Pecan (Pillsbury)	1/12	160	9	51
Chocolate:				
(Duncan Hines)	1/12	160	7	39
(General Foods)	1/12	160	7	39
*Chocolate Chip (Pillsbury)	1/12	150	5	30
Chocolate Fudge (Pillsbury)	1/12	150	6	36
Chocolate, Milk:				
(Duncan Hines)	1/12	155	7	41
(Pillsbury)	1/12	150	6	36
Chocolate Mint (Pillsbury)	1/12	150	7	42
Coconut Almond (Pillsbury)	1/12	150	9	54
Cream Cheese (Pillsbury)	1/12	160	6	34
Dark Chocolate Fudge				
(Duncan Hines)	1/12	155	7	41
Double Dutch (Pillsbury)	1/12	140	6	39
*Lemon (Pillsbury)	1/12	160	2	11
Mocha (Pillsbury)	1/12	150	6	36
Strawberry (Pillsbury)	1/12	160	6	34
Vanilla:				
(Duncan Hines)	1/12	160	7	39
(General Foods)	1/12	160	7	39
(Pillsbury)	1/12	160	6	34
*White Frosting, Fluffy (Pillsbury)	1/12	60	0	0

■ CAKE MIXES

1 SLICE PREPARED ACCORDING TO PACKAGE

Fat Range = 0% to 48%

Average Fat = 28%

FOOD	MEASURE OR QUANTITY	CALORIES	FAT GRAMS	% FAT
Angel Food:				
*(Duncan Hines)	1/12	130	0	0
*(Homemade)	1-1/2 oz	170	0	0
*Angel Food, Chocolate				
(Betty Crocker)	1/12	150	0	0
*Angel Food, Confetti				
(Betty Crocker)	1/12	160	0	0
*Angel Food, Lemon Custard				
(Betty Crocker)	1/12	150	0	0
*Angel Food, Raspberry				
(Betty Crocker)	1/12	140	0	0
*Angel Food, Strawberry				
(Betty Crocker)	1/12	150	0	0
Angel Food, White:				
*(Betty Crocker)	1/12	140	0	0
*(Pillsbury)	1/12	140	0	0
Apple Cinnamon:				
Moist (Betty Crocker)	1/12	260	11	38
*Coffee Cake (Pillsbury)	1/8	240	7	26
Apple, Dutch Streusil (Pillsbury)	1/16	260	11	38
*Applesauce Raisin (Betty Crocker)	1/9	180	4	20

FOOD	MEASURE OR QUANTITY	CALORIES	FAT GRAMS	% FAT
Applesauce Spice (Pillsbury)	1/12	250	11	40
Banana:				
(Betty Crocker)	1/12	260	11	38
(Pillsbury)	1/12	250	11	40
Banana Streusil (Pillsbury)	1/16	260	11	38
*Banana Walnut (Betty Crocker)	1/9	190	6	28
Boston Cream Bundt (Pillsbury)	1/16	270	10	33
Butter Brickle (Betty Crocker)	1/12	260	11	38
Butter Pecan:				
(Betty Crocker)	1/12	250	11	40
*Snackin' Cake (Betty Crocker)	1/9	190	6	28
*Coffee Cake (Pillsbury)	1/8	240	7	26
Butter Streusil (Pillsbury)	1/16	260	11	38
Carrot:				
(Betty Crocker)	1/12	260	12	42
*(Duncan Hines)	1/12	190	4	19
*Carrot with Cream Cheese				
(Betty Crocker)	1/6	230	6	23
*Carrot Nut Snackin' Cake				
(Betty Crocker)	1/9	180	6	30
Carrot and Spice (Pillsbury)	1/12	260	11	38
Cheesecake:				
(Jello-O)	1/8	300	14	42
(Royal Lite)	1/8	210	10	43
*Cherry Chip (Betty Crocker)	1/12	180	3	15
Cherry Supreme (Duncan Hines)	1/12	260	11	38
Chocolate Chip:				
*(Betty Crocker)	1/12	190	4	19
*With Frosting (Betty Crocker)	1/6	230	6	23
Chocolate (Betty Crocker)	1/12	250	12	43
*Chocolate with Frosting				
(Betty Crocker)	1/6	230	6	23
Chocolate (Duncan Hines)	1/12	280	15	48
Chocolate Fudge:				
(Betty Crocker)	1/12	250	11	40
*Fudge (Betty Crocker)	1/9	190	6	28
*With Vanilla Frosting				
(Betty Crocker)	1/6	230	5	20
Chocolate Macaroon Bundt				
(Pillsbury)	1/16	270	12	40
Chocolate Mint (Pillsbury)	1/12	260	12	42
*Chocolate Pudding				
(Betty Crocker)	1/6	230	5	20
Chocolate, German				
(See German Chocolate)				
Chocolate Sour Cream				
(Betty Crocker)	1/12	260	11	38
Chocolate, Swiss				
(Duncan Hines)	1/12	280	15	48
Cinnamon Streusel:				
*Coffee Cake (Pillsbury)	1/8	250	8	29
(Pillsbury)	1/16	260	11	38
Coconut Pecan (Betty Crocker)	1/9	190	7	33
Dark Chocolate Cake (Pillsbury)	1/12	260	12	42
Devil's Food:				
(Betty Crocker)	1/12	270	13	43

FOOD	MEASURE OR QUANTITY	CALORIES	FAT GRAMS	% FAT
*(Duncan Hines)	1/12	190	4	19
(Pillsbury)	1/12	250	11	40
*With Chocolate Frosting				
(Betty Crocker)	1/6	230	6	23
Fudge Bundt (Pillsbury)	1/16	270	12	40
***Fudge Cake** (Duncan Hines)	1/12	185	4	19
Fudge Marble (Pillsbury)	1/12	270	12	40
Fudge Marble Streusil (Pillsbury)	1/16	260	11	38
Fudge Nut Crown Bundt				
(Pillsbury)	1/16	220	9	37
Fudge Peanut Butter Chocolate				
Chip (Betty Crocker)	1/12	200	7	32
German Black Forest (Betty				
Crocker)	1/12	180	7	35
German Chocolate:				
(Betty Crocker)	1/12	260	11	38
*Nut Pecan (Betty Crocker)	1/9	180	5	25
(Pillsbury)	1/12	250	11	40
German Chocolate Streusil:				
*(Betty Crocker)	1/6	240	7	26
(Pillsbury)	1/16	260	11	38
Gingerbread:				
*(Betty Crocker)	1/9	210	7	30
*(Pillsbury)	3" sq	190	4	19
***Golden Cake** (Duncan Hines)	1/12	185	4	19
***Golden Chocolate Chip**				
Snackin' Cake				
(Betty Crocker)	1/9	190	5	24
Lemon:				
(Betty Crocker)	1/12	260	11	38
(Pillsbury)	1/12	260	11	38
Lemon Bluebery Bundt				
(Pillsbury)	1/16	200	8	36
***Lemon Bundt** (Pillsbury)	1/16	270	9	30
***Lemon Chiffon** (Betty Crocker)	1/12	190	4	19
***Lemon Pudding** (Betty Crocker)	1/6	230	5	20
Lemon Streusil (Pillsbury)	1/16	270	11	37
Marble (Betty Crocker)	1/12	260	11	38
Marble Supreme Bundt				
(Pillsbury)	1/16	250	9	32
Milk Chocolate (Betty Crocker)	1/12	250	11	40
***Mint Fudge Chip Snackin' Cake**				
(Betty Crocker)	1/12	190	6	28
Oats 'n Brown Sugar (Pillsbury)	1/12	260	12	42
Orange (Betty Crocker)	1/12	260	11	38
Pecan and Brown Sugar				
Streusil (Pillsbury)	1/16	260	11	38
Pineapple Supreme				
(Duncan Hines)	1/12	260	11	38
Pineapple Upside Down				
(Betty Crocker)	1/9	270	10	33
Pound (Betty Crocker)	1/12	200	9	40
Pound Bundt (Pillsbury)	1/16	230	9	35
Sour Cream Coffee Cake (Pillsbury)	1/8	270	12	40
Spice:				
(Betty Crocker)	1/12	260	11	38

FOOD	MEASURE OR QUANTITY	CALORIES	FAT GRAMS	% FAT
*With Vanilla Frosting (Betty Crocker)	1/6	280	9	29
Strawberry:				
(Betty Crocker)	1/12	260	11	38
(Pillsbury)	1/12	260	11	38
White:				
(Betty Crocker)	1/12	250	10	36
*(Duncan Hines)	1/12	190	4	19
(Pillsbury)	1/12	240	10	38
*White Sour Cream				
(Betty Crocker)	1/12	180	3	15
Yellow:				
*(Duncan Hines)	1/12	190	4	19
(Pillsbury)	1/12	260	12	42
With Chocolate Frosting				
(Betty Crocker)	1/6	230	8	31

■ CAKES AND DANISH, FROZEN

Fat Range = 22% to 81%
Average Fat = 44%

FOOD	MEASURE OR QUANTITY	CALORIES	FAT GRAMS	% FAT
Angel Food (Dolly Madison)	1/6 cake	120	5	38
Apple Danish:				
(Sara Lee)	1	120	6	45
(Store Brand)	5 oz	500	26	47
With Icing (Pillsbury)	1 roll	240	11	41
Apple Fruit Square (Pepperidge Farm)	1	220	12	49
Apple Struedel (Pepperidge Farm)	1	240	10	38
Apple Turnover (Pepperidge Farm)	1	300	17	51
*Banana Cake, One Layer (Sara Lee)	2 oz	150	5	30
Bavarian Cream Puff (Rich's)	1	150	8	48
Black Forest:				
(Sara Lee)	2.5 oz	180	8	40
*(Weight Watchers)	1	180	5	25
Blueberry Fruit Square (Pepperidge Farm)	1	220	11	45
Boston Cream (Pepperidge Farm)	3 oz	290	14	43
Butterscotch Pecan (Pepperidge Farm)	1-5/8 oz	160	7	39
Carrot Cake:				
Cream Cheese Icing (Pepperidge Farm)	1-3/8 oz	140	8	51
One Layer (Sara Lee)	2 oz	260	13	45
(Weight Watchers)	1	170	6	32

FOOD	MEASURE OR QUANTITY	CALORIES	FAT GRAMS	% FAT
Cheese Cake:				
(Sara Lee)	4 oz	350	22	57
*(Weight Watchers)	1	220	7	29
Cheese Danish:				
(Sara Lee)	1	130	8	55
With Icing (Store Brand)	5 oz	600	30	45
Cherry Fruit Square				
(Pepperidge Farm)	1	230	12	47
Cherry Turnover				
(Pepperidge Farm)	1	310	20	58
*Chocolate (Weight Watchers)	1	180	5	25
Chocolate Chip:				
Cheese Cake (Sara Lee)	4 oz	420	27	58
Pound Cake (Sara Lee)	1 oz	130	5	35
Chocolate, Dutch (Pepperidge Farm)	1-¾ oz	190	10	47
Chocolate Fudge Layer				
(Pepperidge Farm)	1-½ oz	180	10	50
Chocolate, German:				
Layer (Pepperidge Farm)	1-½ oz	180	10	50
(Weight Watchers)	1	190	7	33
Chocolate Mint Layer				
(Pepperidge Farm)	1-½ oz	170	9	48
Chocolate Mousse (Sara Lee)	2-¾ oz	250	16	58
Chocolate Supreme				
(Pepperidge Farm)	3 oz	310	17	49
Cinnamon Danish with Icing				
(Pillsbury)	2 rolls	230	9	35
Cinnamon Raisin Danish:				
(Pillsbury)	2 rolls	300	14	42
(Sara Lee)	1	150	8	48
Coconut Layer				
(Pepperidge Farm)	1-½ oz	180	9	45
Danish with Caramel Nuts				
(Pillsbury)	2 rolls	310	16	46
Devil's Food Cake				
(Pepperidge Farm)	1-½ oz	180	9	45
Eclair:				
Regular (Rich's)	1	205	10	44
With Chocolate Icing (Rich's)	1	240	14	52
French Cheese, Lite (Sara Lee)	2 oz	200	13	58
French Cream Cheese Cake				
(Sara Lee)	3 oz	260	17	59
Golden Layer (Pepperidge Farm)	1-½ oz	180	9	45
Grand Marnier				
(Pepperidge Farm)	1-½ oz	190	17	81
Lemon Coconut				
(Pepperidge Farm)	3 oz	280	13	42
Orange Danish with Icing				
(Pillsbury)	1 roll	300	14	42
*Peach Melba				
(Pepperidge Farm)	3 oz	270	7	23
Peach Turnover				
(Pepperidge Farm)	1	310	19	55
Pecan Coffee Cake (Sara Lee)	1-½ oz	160	8	45

FOOD	MEASURE OR QUANTITY	CALORIES	FAT GRAMS	% FAT
Pecan Praline Cheese Cake (Sara Lee)	4 oz	430	30	63
Pineapple Cream (Pepperidge Farm)	2 oz	190	7	33
Pound Cake:				
(Dolly Madison)	1/6 cake	220	8	33
(Pepperidge Farm)	1 oz	130	7	48
(Sara Lee)	1 oz	130	7	48
Snack (Sara Lee)	1-¾ oz	230	12	47
Raspberry Danish (Sara Lee)	1	130	6	42
Raspberry Mocha Cake (Pepperidge Farm)	3 oz	310	14	41
Raspberry Turnover (Pepperidge Farm)	1	310	17	49
Strawberry Cheesecake:				
(Sara Lee)	3.3 oz	250	16	58
*(Weight Watchers)	1	180	5	25
Strawberry Cream Cake (Pepperidge Farm)	2 oz	190	7	33
Strawberry French Cheese Lite (Sara Lee)	2 oz	200	11	50
Strawberry Shortcake:				
(Sara Lee)	2-½ oz	190	8	38
*(Weight Watchers)	1	160	4	22
Vanilla Layer (Pepperidge Farm)	2 oz	190	8	38
Walnut Coffe Cake, (Sara Lee)	1-½ oz	170	9	48
Walnut Raisin Pound Cake (Sara Lee)	1-½ oz	140	5	32

■ PIES, FROZEN

10-INCH PIE CUT INTO 8 SLICES
Fat Range = 27% to 56%
Average Fat = 40%

FOOD	MEASURE OR QUANTITY	CALORIES	FAT GRAMS	% FAT
Apple:				
Lattice (Mrs. Smith)	⅛ pie	350	13	33
Old Fashioned (Mrs. Smith)	⅛ pie	515	27	47
(Mrs. Smith)	⅛ pie	390	17	39
Banana Cream (Mrs. Smith)	⅛ pie	240	12	45
Blueberry (Mrs. Smith)	⅛ pie	380	17	40
*Boston Cream (Mrs. Smith)	⅛ pie	260	8	28
Cherry:				
(Mrs. Smith)	⅛ pie	400	18	41
*Lattice (Mrs. Smith)	⅛ pie	350	11	28
Chocolate Cream (Mrs. Smith)	⅛ pie	270	13	43
Coconut Cream (Mrs. Smith)	⅛ pie	270	14	47
Coconut Custard (Mrs. Smith)	⅛ pie	330	15	41
*Egg Custard (Mrs. Smith)	⅛ pie	300	9	27
Lemon Cream (Mrs. Smith)	⅛ pie	245	12	44
*Lemon Meringue (Mrs. Smith)	⅛ pie	310	10	29

FOOD	MEASURE OR QUANTITY	CALORIES	FAT GRAMS	% FAT
Peach (Mrs. Smith)	⅛ pie	365	16	39
Pecan (Mrs. Smith)	⅛ pie	500	23	41
Pie Crust Shell:				
(Mrs. Smith)	⅛ pie	130	8	55
(Pillsbury)	⅛ pie	240	15	56
Pumpkin (Mrs. Smith)	⅛ pie	300	11	33

■ PIES, HOMEMADE
10-INCH PIE CUT INTO 8 SLICES
Fat Range = 29% to 58%
Average Fat = 40%

FOOD	MEASURE OR QUANTITY	CALORIES	FAT GRAMS	% FAT
Apple	⅛ pie	300	12	36
Banana Cream	⅛ pie	250	11	40
Blackberry	⅛ pie	290	12	37
Blueberry	⅛ pie	300	12	36
*Boston Cream	⅛ pie	250	8	29
Cherry	⅛ pie	300	14	42
Chocolate Cream	⅛ pie	300	15	45
Coconut Custard	⅛ pie	300	14	42
Lemon Meringue	⅛ pie	350	13	33
Peach	⅛ pie	300	12	36
Pecan	⅛ pie	450	25	50
Pie Crust	1 shell	1000	65	58
Pineapple	⅛ pie	300	13	39
Pineapple Custard	⅛ pie	250	10	36
Pumpkin	⅛ pie	260	14	48
Rhubarb	⅛ pie	300	14	42
Strawberry	⅛ pie	200	7	32

■ PIES, READY-TO-EAT
Fat Range = 21% to 52%
Average Fat = 37%

FOOD	MEASURE OR QUANTITY	CALORIES	FAT GRAMS	% FAT
Apple:				
(Drakes)	1	220	10	41
(Hostess)	1	400	20	45
(McDonald's)	1	260	15	52
(Tastycake)	1	345	12	31
*(Weight Watcher's)	1	190	5	24
*Apple, French (Tastycake)	1	400	13	29
Berry (Hostess)	1	390	20	46
Blueberry (Hostess)	1	390	20	46

FOOD	MEASURE OR QUANTITY	CALORIES	FAT GRAMS	% FAT
*Boston Cream				
(Weight Watcher's)	1	170	4	21
Cherry:				
(Hostess)	1	390	20	46
(Tastycake)	1	370	13	32
Chocolate Pudding (Tastycake)	1	440	16	33
Coconut Cream (Tastycake)	1	430	22	46
Lemon:				
Hostess	1	400	21	47
Lemon (Tastycake)	1	360	13	32
Peach:				
(Hostess)	1	400	22	50
(Tastycake)	1	340	12	32
*Pineapple (Tastycake)	1	360	12	30
*Pudding (Hostess)	1	470	13	25
Pumpkin (Tastycake)	1	360	14	35
Strawberry:				
(Hostess)	1	340	14	37
*(Tastycake)	1	370	12	29
Tasty Klair (Tastycake)	1	435	19	39
Vanilla Pudding (Tastycake)	1	430	19	40

■ PUDDINGS AND PIE FILLINGS

PREPARED WITH WHOLE MILK AS PACKAGE DIRECTS

Fat Range = 0% to 35%

Average Fat = 22%

FOOD	MEASURE OR QUANTITY	CALORIES	FAT GRAMS	% FAT
Banana Cream:				
*(Jell-O)	4 oz	170	5	26
*(Royal)	4 oz	160	4	22
*Pie Filling (Jell-O)	1/6	100	3	27
*Butter Almond (Royal)	4 oz	170	4	21
*Butter Pecan (Jell-O)	4 oz	170	5	26
Butterscotch:				
*(Del Monte)	5 oz	180	5	25
*(D-Zerta)[1]	4 oz	70	0	0
*(Jell-O)	5 oz	170	4	21
Butterscotch, Sugar Free:				
*(Jell-O)[2]	4 oz	90	2	20
*(Royal)[2]	4 oz	100	2	18
Chocolate:				
*(Del Monte)	5 oz	190	6	28
*(D-Zerta)[1]	4 oz	60	0	0
*(Jell-O)	4 oz	160	4	22
*(Junket)	5 oz	120	4	30
*(Royal)	4 oz	180	4	20

[1]Prepared with skim milk.
[2]Prepared with two percent milk.

FOOD	MEASURE OR QUANTITY	CALORIES	FAT GRAMS	% FAT
*Chocolate Chip (Royal)	4 oz	190	4	19
Chocolate Fudge:				
*(Del Monte)	5 oz	190	6	28
*(Jell-O)	4 oz	160	4	22
*Chocolate, Milk (Jell-O)	4 oz	170	4	21
*Chocolate, Mint (Royal)	4 oz	190	4	19
Chocolate, Sugar Free:				
*(Jell-O)[2]	4 oz	100	3	27
*(Royal)[2]	4 oz	110	3	25
Coconut Cream:				
(Jell-O)	4 oz	180	7	35
Pie Filling (Jell-O)	1/6	110	4	33
*Coconut Custard (Royal)	4 oz	150	5	30
*Egg Custard, Golden (Jell-O)	4 oz	160	5	28
*Key Lime (Royal)	4 oz	160	3	17
Lemon:				
*(Jell-O)	4 oz	180	4	20
*(Royal)	4 oz	180	5	25
*Pie Filling (Jell-O)	1/6	170	2	11
*Pineapple Cream (Jell-O)	4 oz	170	4	21
Pistachio:				
*(Jell-O)	4 oz	180	5	25
*(Royal)	4 oz	170	4	21
*Rice (Jell-O)	4 oz	170	4	21
*Tapioca, Chocolate (Jell-O)	4 oz	170	5	26
Vanilla:				
*(Del Monte)	5 oz	180	5	25
*(D-Zerta)[1]	4 oz	70	0	0
*(Jell-O)	4 oz	160	4	22
*(Junket)	5 oz	120	4	30
*(Royal)	4 oz	160	1	6
*Vanilla, French (Jell-O)	4 oz	170	4	21
Vanilla, Sugar Free:				
*(Jell-O)[2]	4 oz	90	2	20
*(Royal)[2]	4 oz	100	2	18

■ PUDDINGS, READY-TO-EAT
Fat Range = 20% to 49%
Average Fat = 34%

FOOD	MEASURE OR QUANTITY	CALORIES	FAT GRAMS	% FAT
Banana:				
*(Del Monte)	5 oz	180	5	25
(Hunt's)	5 oz	210	11	47
Butterscotch:				
*(Del Monte)	5 oz	180	5	25

[1] Prepared with skim milk
[2] Prepared with two percent milk.

FOOD	MEASURE OR QUANTITY	CALORIES	FAT GRAMS	% FAT
(Hunt's)	5 oz	210	9	39
(Swiss Miss)	4 oz	140	6	39
Chocolate:				
*(Del Monte)	5 oz	190	6	28
(Hunt's)	5 oz	210	9	39
(Swiss Miss)	4 oz	150	6	36
Chocolate Fudge:				
*(Del Monte)	5 oz	190	6	28
(Hunt's)	5 oz	200	10	45
(Swiss Miss)	4 oz	170	6	32
Chocolate, German (Hunt's)	5 oz	220	9	37
*Lemon (Hunt's)	5 oz	180	4	20
Marshmallow (Hunt's)	5 oz	200	9	40
Rice (Hunt's)	5 oz	220	12	49
Tapioca:				
*(Del Monte)	5 oz	180	4	20
(Hunt's)	5 oz	140	6	39
*(Swiss Miss)	4 oz	130	4	28
Vanilla:				
*(Del Monte)	5 oz	180	5	25
(Hunt's)	5 oz	210	9	39
(Swiss Miss)	4 oz	140	6	39
Vanilla with Fudge (Swiss Miss)	4 oz	160	7	39

■ SNACK CAKES, PACKAGED

Fat Range = 0% to 63%
Average Fat = 34%

FOOD	MEASURE OR QUANTITY	CALORIES	FAT GRAMS	% FAT
*Allspice, Lights (Hostess)	1	130	1	7
*Apple Delights (Little Debbie)	1 pkg	140	4	26
Apple, Dutch (Little Debbie)	1 pkg	230	8	31
*Banana Crunch Cake, Fat Free				
(Entemann's)	1 oz	80	0	0
Banana Slices (Little Debbie)	1 pkg	340	12	32
*Banana Treats (Tastycake)	1	150	4	24
Big Wheels (Hostess)	1	170	9	48
Carrot Cake, Deluxe (Sara Lee)	1	180	7	35
Cheesecake, Classic (Sara Lee)	1	200	14	63
Cheesecake, French Strawberry (Sara Lee)	1	200	13	58
Chip Flips (Hostess)	1	330	16	44
Choco-Diles (Hostess)	1	240	11	41
Choc-O-Jel (Little Debbie)	1	150	7	42
Chocolate:				
*Chocolate Filled, Lights (Hostess)	1	110	1	8
*Raspberry Filled, Lights (Hostess)	1	130	1	7
*Vanilla Pudding Filled Lights (Hostess)	1	140	1	6

FOOD	MEASURE OR QUANTITY	CALORIES	FAT GRAMS	% FAT
Chocolate Fudge Cake				
(Sara Lee)	1	190	10	47
Chocolate Holiday Cakes				
(Little Debbie)	1 pkg	320	15	42
Chocolate Snack Cakes				
(Little Debbie)	1 pkg	390	19	44
Christmas Trees (Little Debbie)	1 pkg	220	11	45
*Coconut Crunch (Little Debbie)	1 pkg	320	9	25
Coconut Rounds (Little Debbie)	1 pkg	150	7	42
*Coconut Twins (Little Debbie)	1 pkg	240	7	26
Coffee Cake:				
Butter and Cinnamon				
(Sara Lee)	1	290	13	40
Cinnamon (Sara Lee)	1	290	13	40
*Cinnamon Apple Fat Free				
(Entemann's)	1 oz	90	0	0
(Drake's)	1	140	6	39
Pecan (Sara Lee)	1	280	16	51
Streusil (Sara Lee)	1	230	12	47
*Creamie (Tastycake)	1	195	2	9
Crumb Cake (Hostess)	1	150	8	48
Cupcake, Chocolate:				
(Homemade)	1	130	5	35
(Hostess)	1	170	6	32
(Tastycake)	1	113	4	32
Cupcake, Chocolate Chip				
(Homemade)	1	180	7	35
Cupcake, Chocolate Filled				
(Tastycake)	1	138	6	39
Cupcake, Creme Filled				
(Tastycake)	1	130	5	35
*Cupcake, Orange (Hostess)	1	150	5	30
Cupcake, Vanilla:				
(Homemade)	1	120	5	38
(Tastycake)	1	116	5	39
Cupcake with Vanilla Icing				
(Homemade)	1	170	7	37
Dessert Cups:				
*(Hostess)	1	60	0	0
*(Little Debbie)	1 pkg	80	1	11
*Devil Creams (Little Debbie)	1 pkg	320	9	25
Devil Dogs (Drake's)	1	170	8	42
Devil Squares (Little Debbie)	1 pkg	270	11	37
Ding Dong (Hostess)	1	170	9	48
Easter Bunny Cake (Little				
Debbie)	1 pkg	320	15	42
Fancy Cakes (Little Debbie)	1 pkg	340	16	42
*Figaroos (Little Debbie)	1 pkg	160	4	22
Fudge Bar (Tastycake)	1	266	11	37
*Fudge Crispy (Little Debbie)	1 pkg	260	7	24
Fudge Rounds (Little Debbie)	1 pkg	150	6	36
Funny Bones (Drakes)	1	160	9	51
Golden Cremes (Little Debbie)	1 pkg	270	11	37
*Golden Loaf Fat Free				
(Entemann's)	1 oz	80	0	0
Ho-Hos (Hostess)	1	120	6	45

FOOD	MEASURE OR QUANTITY	CALORIES	FAT GRAMS	% FAT
Honeybuns, Glazed (Tastycake)	1	330	13	35
Hostess O's (Hostess)	1	240	11	41
*Ice Cream Cups (Little Debbie)	1 pkg	15	0	0
*Jelly Krimpets (Tastycake)	1	112	2	16
Jelly Rolls (Little Debbie)	1 pkg	250	9	32
*Junior Orange (Tastycake)	1	350	11	28
Junior (Tastycake)	1	350	12	31
Kandy Kane (Tastycake)	1	106	5	42
Koffee Kake (Tastycake)	1	330	12	33
Kreme Cups (Tastycake)	1	115	5	39
Krimpets (Tastycake)	1	130	5	35
Lemon Stix (Little Debbie)	1 pkg	220	10	41
*Light's Apple Spice (Hostess)	1	130	1	7
*Li'l Angels (Hostess)	1	90	2	20
Marshmallow Sup (Little Debbie)	1 pkg	130	5	35
Mint Sprints (Little Debbie)	1 pkg	200	10	45
Nutty Bar (Little Debbie)	1 pkg	310	20	58
Nutty Wafers (Little Debbie)	1 pkg	310	20	58
*Oatmeal Raisin Bar (Tastycake)	1	240	8	30
Peanut Butter Bar (Little Debbie)	1 pkg	260	13	45
Peanut Clusters (Little Debbie)	1 pkg	220	11	45
Peanut Putters (Hostess)	1	410	21	46
Pecan Twins (Little Debbie)	1 pkg	220	10	41
*Pineapple Crunch Cake Fat Free (Entemann's)	1 oz	70	0	0
Pound Cake:				
All Butter (Sara Lee)	1	200	11	50
Regular (Sara Lee)	1	210	12	51
Pumpkin Delights (Little Debbie)	1 pkg	140	6	39
Ring Ding (Drake's)	1	160	9	51
*Sno-Balls (Hostess)	1	150	4	24
Spice Cakes (Little Debbie)	1 pkg	270	11	37
Star Crunch (Little Debbie)	1 pkg	150	6	36
Suzy Q's (Hostess)	1	240	9	34
Swiss Cake Roll (Little Debbie)	1 pkg	270	12	40
Tempty (Tastycakes)	1	97	4	37
*Tiger Tails (Hostess)	1	210	6	26
Toastettes (See Toaster Cakes)				
*Twinkies (Hostess)	1	160	5	28
Vanilla Snack Cake (Little Debbie)	1 pkg	330	16	44
Yankee Doodles (Drake's)	1	110	5	41
Yodels (Drake's)	1	115	5	39

9. EGGS

■ EGGS, EGG SUBSTITUTES,
EGG DISHES, AND QUICHES
Fat Range = 0% to 82%
Average Fat = 56%

FOOD	MEASURE OR QUANTITY	CALORIES	FAT GRAMS	% FAT
Country Morning				
(Land O' Lakes)	4 oz	173	12	62
Egg Beaters (Fleischmann's)				
*Plain	2 oz	25	0	0
With Cheese	2 oz	130	6	42
Egg, Chicken:				
Extra Large	1	90	6	60
Fried in Butter	1	91	7	69
Hard Boiled	1	82	6	66
Jumbo	1	100	7	63
Large	1	82	6	66
Poached	1	80	6	68
Scrambled in Milk and Butter:				
1 egg	1	108	8	67
2 eggs	1	130	10	69
*White	1 cup	120	0	0
*White	1	12	0	0
Egg-Yolk	1	66	6	82
Egg, Duck,	1	130	10	69
Egg, Goose	1	270	20	67
***Egg Powder**	1 oz	130	4	28
Egg, Quail	1	14	1	64
Egg Substitute:				
Frozen	2 oz	96	7	66
Liquid	2 oz	50	3	54
Egg, Turkey	1	135	9	60
Omelet:				
Cheese and Mushroom, 2 Eggs	1	250	17	61
Ham and Cheese (Swanson)	7 oz	400	31	70
Spanish (Swanson)	7-¾ oz	250	17	61
Western:				
*(Durkee)	1	170	5	26
2 Eggs (Homemade)	1	170	6	32
Quiche:				
Bacon & Onion (Pour-a-Quiche)	4 oz	230	18	70
Ham (Pour-a-Quiche)	4 oz	230	17	67
Spinach and Onion				
(Pour-a-Quiche)	4 oz	220	16	65
Scrambled:				
(Durkee)	1	125	10	72
(Land O' Lakes)	4 oz	143	9	57

FOOD	MEASURE OR QUANTITY	CALORIES	FAT GRAMS	% FAT
With Bacon (Durkee)	1	181	13	65
With Sausage and Hash Browns (Swanson)	6 oz	410	33	72
*Scramblers (Morningstar)	2 oz	60	2	30
Souffle:				
Cheese (Homemade)	1 cup	220	17	70
Spinach (Homemade)	1 cup	210	15	64

10. FAST-FOOD RESTAURANTS

■ ARBY'S
Fat Range = 0% to 69%
Fat Average = 34%

FOOD	MEASURE OR QUANTITY	CALORIES	FAT GRAMS	% FAT
Chicken Breast:				
*Roasted	1	254	7	25
Sandwich	1	592	27	41
Chicken Club	1	621	32	46
Chicken Leg	1	319	16	45
Chicken Salad Sandwich	1	386	20	46
Chicken Salad and Croissant:				
Plain	1	472	36	69
With Tomato	1	515	36	63
French Fries	1	246	14	51
Ham 'n Cheese, Hot	1	353	13	33
Hamburger:				
Bac'n Cheddar Deluxe	1	561	34	55
Beef'n Cheddar	1	490	21	39
Potato, Baked:				
*Plain	1	290	0	0
With Broccoli and Cheese	1	541	22	37
Potato Cakes	2	201	14	63
With Mushroom and Cheese	1	506	22	39
Superstuff	1	648	38	53
***Rice Pilaf**	1	123	2	15
Roast Beef:				
Deluxe	1	486	23	43
Junior	1	218	8	33
King	1	467	19	37
Regular	1	350	15	39
Super	1	501	22	40
***Salad, Tossed, Plain**	1	44	0	0

FOOD	MEASURE OR QUANTITY	CALORIES	FAT GRAMS	% FAT
Shake:				
*(Chocolate)	1	384	11	26
*(Jamocha)	1	424	10	21
(Vanilla)	1	295	10	31
Taco	1	619	27	39
Turkey Deluxe	1	375	17	41
Vegetables and Sauce	1	56	2	32

■ **ARTHUR TREACHER'S SEAFOOD RESTAURANT**
Fat Range = 23% to 59%
Average Fat = 43%

FOOD	MEASURE OR QUANTITY	CALORIES	FAT GRAMS	% FAT
Bake 'n Broil, Cod Tail	1	245	14	51
Chicken:				
Piece	1	370	22	54
*Sandwich	1	420	12	26
Chips	1	276	13	42
Cole Slaw	1	123	8	59
Fish:				
Piece	1	355	20	50
Sandwich	1	440	24	49
Lemon Luvs	1	276	14	46
Shrimp	1	380	24	57

■ **BURGER KING**
Fat Range = 0% to 93%
Average Fat = 47%

FOOD	MEASURE OR QUANTITY	CALORIES	FAT GRAMS	% FAT
Apple Pie	1	305	12	35
Breakfast Croissantwich:				
Bacon, Egg and Cheese	1	355	24	61
Egg and Sausage	1	335	20	54
Sausage, Egg and Cheese	1	538	41	69
Cheeseburger:				
Regular	1	317	15	43
Double:				
Bacon	1	510	31	55
Bacon Deluxe	1	592	39	59
Mushroom Swiss	1	473	27	51
Regular	1	483	27	50
Cherry Pie	1	357	13	33
Chicken, *BK Broiler*	1	380	18	43
Chicken Sandwich	1	688	40	52
Chicken Tenders	6	236	13	50

FOOD	MEASURE OR QUANTITY	CALORIES	FAT GRAMS	% FAT
Egg:				
With Bacon	1	536	36	60
With Sausage	1	702	52	67
Egg Platter	1	468	30	58
Fish Tenders	6	267	16	54
French Fries	1	227	13	52
French Toast:				
With Bacon	1	469	30	58
With Sausage	1	635	46	65
Ham and Cheese Sandwich	1	471	23	44
Hamburger	1	275	12	39
Onion Rings	1	274	16	53
Pecan Pie	1	459	20	39
Ranch Dipping Sauce	1	171	18	95
Salad Dressing:				
Blue Cheese	1	184	16	78
Creamy Italian	1	170	15	79
French	1	152	11	65
House Dressing	1	159	13	74
Italian	1	162	14	78
*Low Calorie	1	42	1	21
1000 Island	1	145	12	74
*Salad, Plain	1	28	0	0
Shake:				
Chocolate Medium	1	320	12	34
*Vanilla Medium	1	321	10	28
*Sweet and Sour Dipping Sauce	1	45	0	0
Tartar Dipping Sauce	1	174	18	93
Tater Tenders	1	213	12	51
Whaler:				
Regular	1	488	27	50
With Cheese	1	530	30	51
Whopper:				
Regular	1	640	41	58
With Cheese	1	723	48	60
***Whopper* Double:**				
Regular	1	850	52	55
With Cheese	1	950	60	57
***Whopper* Junior:**				
Regular	1	370	17	41
With Cheese	1	420	20	43

■ **CHURCH'S**
   Fat Range = 0% to 76%
   Average Fat = 40%

FOOD	MEASURE OR QUANTITY	CALORIES	FAT GRAMS	% FAT
Cole Slaw	1	83	7	76
*Corn Cob	1	165	3	16

FOOD	MEASURE OR QUANTITY	CALORIES	FAT GRAMS	% FAT
Crispy Nuggets:				
Regular	1	55	3	49
Spicy	1	52	3	52
*Dinner Roll	1	83	2	22
French Fries	1	256	13	46
Fried Chicken:				
Breast	1	278	17	55
Leg	1	147	9	55
Thigh	1	306	22	65
Wing and Breast	1	303	20	59
Hush Puppies	1	78	3	35
*Jalapeño Pepper	1	4	0	0
Pecan Pie	1	367	20	49
Southern Fried Catfish	1	67	4	54

■ **DAIRY QUEEN**
Fat Range = 0% to 57%
Average Fat = 30%

FOOD	MEASURE OR QUANTITY	CALORIES	FAT GRAMS	% FAT
*Banana Split	1	540	11	18
Buster Bar	1	460	29	57
Chicken Sandwich	1	670	41	55
Cone:				
*Large	1	340	10	26
*Regular	1	240	7	26
*Small	1	140	4	26
Cone, Dipped:				
Large	1	510	24	42
Regular	1	340	16	42
Small	1	190	9	43
Dilly Bar	1	210	13	56
Double Delight	1	490	20	37
**D Q Sandwich*	1	140	4	26
Fish Sandwich:				
Regular	1	400	17	38
With Cheese	1	440	21	43
*Float	1	410	7	15
*Freeze	1	500	12	22
French Fries:				
Large	1	320	16	45
Small	1	200	10	45
Hamburger, Double:				
Regular	1	530	28	48
With Cheese	1	650	37	51
Hamburger, Single:				
Regular	1	360	16	40
With Cheese	1	410	20	44

FOOD	MEASURE OR QUANTITY	CALORIES	FAT GRAMS	% FAT
Hamburger, Triple:				
Regular	1	710	45	57
With Cheese	1	820	50	55
Hot Dog:				
Regular	1	280	16	51
With Cheese	1	330	21	57
With Chili	1	320	20	56
Hot Dog, Super:				
Regular	1	520	27	47
With Cheese	1	580	34	53
With Chili	1	570	32	51
Hot Fudge Brownie	1	600	25	38
Malt:				
*Large	1	1060	25	21
*Regular	1	760	18	21
*Small	1	520	13	22
Mr. Misty:				
*Float	1	390	7	16
*Freeze	1	500	12	22
*Kiss	1	70	0	0
Plain:				
*Large	1	340	0	0
*Regular	1	250	0	0
*Small	1	190	0	0
Onion Rings	1	280	16	51
***Parfait**	1	430	8	17
Peanut Buster Parfait	1	740	34	41
Shake:				
*Large	1	990	26	24
*Regular	1	710	19	24
*Small	1	490	13	24
***Strawberry Shortcake**	1	540	11	18
Sundae:				
*Large	1	440	10	20
*Regular	1	310	8	23
*Small	1	190	4	19

■ DOMINO'S PIZZA
Fat Range = 21% to 41%
Average Fat = 30%
Each Serving Equals 2 Slices

FOOD	MEASURE OR QUANTITY	CALORIES	FAT GRAMS	% FAT
***Cheese**	2	376	10	24
Deluxe	2	500	20	36
Double Cheese with Pepperoni	2	545	25	41
***Ham**	2	420	11	24
Pepperoni	2	460	18	35
Sausage with Mushroom	2	430	16	33
Veggie	2	500	19	34

■ HARDEE'S
Fat Range = 20% to 49%
Average Fat = 42%

FOOD	MEASURE OR QUANTITY	CALORIES	FAT GRAMS	% FAT
Biscuit:				
Bacon and Egg	1	405	26	58
Ham	1	349	17	44
Ham and Egg	1	458	26	51
Sausage	1	413	26	57
Sausage and Egg	1	521	35	60
Steak	1	419	23	49
Steak and Egg	1	527	31	53
Cheeseburger:				
Bacon	1	686	42	55
Quarter Pound	1	506	26	46
Regular	1	335	17	46
Chicken Fillet	1	510	26	46
Fisherman's Fillet	1	514	26	46
French Fries:				
Large	1	381	21	50
Small	1	239	13	49
Ham and Cheese Hot	1	376	15	36
Hamburger:				
Big Deluxe	1	546	26	43
Regular	1	305	13	38
Hot Dog	1	346	22	57
***Milkshake**	1	391	10	23
Roast Beef Sandwich:				
Regular	1	377	17	41
Big	1	418	19	41
Turnover, Apple	1	282	14	45

■ KENTUCKY FRIED CHICKEN
Fat Range = 14% to 67%
Average Fat = 44%

FOOD	MEASURE OR QUANTITY	CALORIES	FAT GRAMS	% FAT
***Baked Beans**	1	105	2	17
Biscuit	1	235	12	46
Chicken, Extra Crispy:				
Breast	1	340	20	53
Drumstick	1	204	14	62
Thigh	1	406	30	67
Wing	1	254	18	64
Chicken Little's Sandwich	1	170	10	53
Chicken Nugget	1	46	3	59
Chicken, Original Recipe:				
Breast	1	280	16	51
Drumstick	1	147	9	55

FOOD	MEASURE OR QUANTITY	CALORIES	FAT GRAMS	% FAT
Thigh	1	295	19	58
Wing	1	181	12	60
Cole Slaw	1	120	7	52
Colonel's Chicken Sandwich	1	482	27	50
*Corn Cob	1	176	3	15
Kentucky Fries	1	245	12	44
*Potato, Mashed and Gravy	1	71	2	25
Potato Salad	1	141	9	57

■ LONG JOHN SILVER'S RESTAURANT
Fat Range = 36% to 47%
Average Fat = 38%

FOOD	MEASURE OR QUANTITY	CALORIES	FAT GRAMS	% FAT
Chicken Plank, Fryes and Hushpuppy	Kid Meal	510	24	42
Chicken Plank Dinner	4 pieces	940	44	42
Chicken Plank Dinner	3 pieces	830	39	42
Clam Dinner	1	980	45	41
Fish and Chicken Dinner	1	870	40	41
Fish and Fryes	2 pieces	660	30	41
Fish and Fryes	3 pieces	810	38	42
Fish and More	1	800	37	42
Fish Dinner	3 pieces	960	44	41
Fish, Fryes & Hushpuppy	Kid Meal	440	20	41
Fish, Plank and Fryes	Kid Meal	550	26	43
Seafood Platter	1	970	46	43
Shrimp Dinner	6 pieces	740	37	45
Shrimp Dinner	9 pieces	860	45	47
Shrimp, Fish and Chicken Dinner	1	840	40	43

■ MCDONALD'S
Fat Range = 18% to 80%
Average Fat = 40%

FOOD	MEASURE OR QUANTITY	CALORIES	FAT GRAMS	% FAT
Apple Danish	1	390	18	42
Apple Pie	1	253	14	50
Big Mac	1	570	35	55
Biscuit:				
Egg, Bacon and Cheese	1	440	27	55
Sausage and Egg	1	520	34	59
Cheese Danish	1	390	22	51
Cheeseburger	1	310	14	41

FOOD	MEASURE OR QUANTITY	CALORIES	FAT GRAMS	% FAT
Cherry Pie	1	260	14	48
Chicken McNuggets	1	323	21	59
Cinnamon Raisin Danish	1	440	21	43
Cookies	1	308	11	32
Cookies, Chocolate Chip	1	342	16	42
Egg McMuffin	1	290	11	34
Eggs, Scrambled	1	180	13	65
*English Muffin, Buttered	1	186	5	24
Filet-o-Fish	1	435	26	54
French Fries, Regular	1	220	12	49
Hamburger	1	263	11	38
Hash Browns	1	130	7	48
*Hot Cakes with Syrup	1	410	9	20
Mc Chicken	1	490	29	53
Mc DLT	1	680	44	58
Pork Sausage	1	180	16	80
Quarter Pounder:				
Regular	1	427	23	48
With Cheese	1	525	31	53
Raspberry Danish	1	410	16	35
Sausage	1	210	18	77
Sausage McMuffin:				
Regular	1	370	21	51
With Egg	1	440	26	53
Shake:				
*Chocolate	1	383	9	21
*Strawberry	1	362	9	22
*Vanilla	1	352	8	20
Sundae:				
*Caramel	1	360	10	25
*Hot Fudge	1	360	11	28
*Strawberry	1	320	9	25

■ PIZZA HUT
Fat Range = 29% to 46%
Average Fat = 36%
Serving Equals 2 Slices of Medium Pizza

FOOD	MEASURE OR QUANTITY	CALORIES	FAT GRAMS	% FAT
Hand Tossed:				
Cheese	1	518	20	35
Pepperoni	1	500	23	41
Supreme	1	540	26	43
Super Supreme	1	560	25	40
Pan Pizza:				
Cheese	1	492	18	33
Pepperoni	1	540	22	37
Supreme	1	590	30	46
Super Supreme	1	560	26	42

FOOD	MEASURE OR QUANTITY	CALORIES	FAT GRAMS	% FAT
Personal Pan:				
Pepperoni	1 pie	675	29	39
Supreme	1 pie	650	28	39
Thin 'n Crispy:				
Cheese	1	400	17	38
Pepperoni	1	413	20	44
Supreme	1	459	22	43
Super Supreme	1	460	21	41

■ **ROY ROGERS**
Fat Range = 0% to 78%
Average Fat = 41%

FOOD	MEASURE OR QUANTITY	CALORIES	FAT GRAMS	% FAT
Bar Burger	1	610	39	58
Biscuit	1	230	12	47
Breakfast Crescent Sandwich:				
Regular	1	400	25	56
With Bacon	1	435	32	66
With Ham	1 oz	560	45	72
With Sausage	1	450	30	60
*Broccoli	1	40	0	0
Brownie	1	270	11	37
Cheeseburger:				
Regular	1	560	37	59
With Bacon	1	580	39	61
Cheese, Cheddar	1 oz	115	10	78
Chicken:				
Breast	1	330	20	55
Breast and Wing	1	470	30	57
Leg	1	120	8	60
Thigh	1	280	20	64
Thigh and Leg	1	400	26	58
Wing	1	140	10	64
Cole Slaw	3 oz	110	8	65
Crescent Roll	1	290	18	56
Danish:				
Apple	1	250	12	43
Cheese	1	250	11	40
Cherry	1	270	14	47
Egg Platter:				
With Bacon and Biscuit	1	435	30	62
With Biscuit	1	400	30	68
With Ham and Biscuit	1	440	29	59
With Sausage and Biscuit	1	550	40	65
French Fries:				
Large	1	360	18	45
Regular	1	270	14	47
Hamburger	1	455	28	55
Pancake Platter:				
*Regular	1	460	15	29

FOOD	MEASURE OR QUANTITY	CALORIES	FAT GRAMS	% FAT
With Bacon	1	500	18	32
*With Ham	1	510	17	30
With Sausage	1	610	30	44
Potato:				
*Plain	1	200	0	0
With Bacon and Cheese	1	400	22	50
*With Butter	1	280	7	22
With Broccoli and Cheese	1	380	18	43
With Sour Cream and Chives	1	408	20	44
With Taco Beef and Cheese	1	463	22	43
Potato Salad	3 oz	100	6	54
Roast Beef Sandwich:				
*Large	1	360	12	30
*Regular	1	317	10	28
With Cheese Sauce	1	425	19	40
Shake:				
*Chocolate	1	360	10	25
*Strawberry	1	315	10	29
Vanilla	1	305	11	32
Strawberry Shortcake	1	450	19	38
Sundae:				
*Caramel	1	300	8	24
Hot Fudge	1	340	13	34
*Strawberry	1	220	7	29

■ TACO BELL
Fat Range = 23% to 61%
Average Fat = 40%

FOOD	MEASURE OR QUANTITY	CALORIES	FAT GRAMS	% FAT
Burrito:				
Bean:				
*With Green Sauce	1	350	10	26
*With Red Sauce	1	355	10	25
Beef:				
With Green Sauce	1	400	17	38
With Red Sauce	1	390	17	39
Double Beef:				
With Red Sauce	1	460	21	41
Supreme with Green Sauce	1	450	21	42
Supreme:				
With Green Sauce	1	410	18	40
With Red Sauce	1	412	18	39
Chicken Fajita	1	225	11	44
Cinnamon Crispas	1	260	15	52
Enchirito:				
With Green Sauce	1	370	19	46
With Red Sauce	1	380	19	45
Mexican Pizza	1	575	36	56

FOOD	MEASURE OR QUANTITY	CALORIES	FAT GRAMS	% FAT
Nachos:				
Bellgrande	1	650	35	48
Regular	1	350	18	46
Pintos and Cheese:				
With Green Sauce	1	184	8	39
With Red Sauce	1	190	8	38
Steak Fajita	1	233	11	42
Taco:				
Bellgrande	1	355	23	58
Light	1	410	28	61
Regular	1	180	10	50
Super Combo	1	285	16	51
Taco Salad:				
With Salsa	1	940	61	58
With Salsa, without Shell	1	520	31	54
Without Shell	1	500	31	56
Taco, Soft:				
Regular	1	230	11	43
Supreme	1	275	16	52
Tostada:				
With Green Sauce	1	235	11	42
With Red Sauce	1	240	11	41

■ **WENDY'S**
Fat Range = 0% to 96%
Average Fat = 45%

FOOD	MEASURE OR QUANTITY	CALORIES	FAT GRAMS	% FAT
Blue Cheese, dressing	1	90	9	90
Breakfast Sandwich	1	370	19	46
Butterscotch Pudding	1	90	4	40
Cheeseburger:				
Bacon	1	460	28	55
Kids Meal	1	320	15	42
Small	1	320	15	42
Chef Salad	1	180	9	45
Chicken Fried Steak	1	580	41	64
Chicken Sandwich	1	430	19	40
***Chili**	8 oz	260	8	28
Chili, New	1	230	9	35
Chocolate Pudding	1	90	4	40
Cole Slaw	1	60	6	90
Creamy Peppercorn, dressing	1	80	8	90
Crispy Chicken Nuggets	6	290	21	65
Fish Fillet	1	210	11	47
French Fries, Regular	1	280	14	45
French Toast, 2 slices	1	400	19	43
Frosty Dessert	1	400	14	32
Hamburger:				
Bacon Swiss	1	710	44	56
Big Classic	1	580	34	53

FOOD	MEASURE OR QUANTITY	CALORIES	FAT GRAMS	% FAT
Classic with Cheese	1	640	40	56
Double	1	560	34	55
Kids Meal	1	260	9	31
Philly Swiss	1	510	24	42
*Single	1	260	9	23
With Cheese	1	490	28	51
With Everything	1	430	22	46
Without Bun	¼ lb.	210	14	60
Hidden Valley Ranch, dressing	1	50	5	96
Home Fries	1	360	22	55
Italian Dressing:				
Reduced	1	25	2	35
Golden	1	50	4	61
Omelet:				
Cheese and Onion	1	280	19	61
Cheese with Mushrooms	1	290	21	65
Ham and Cheese	1	250	17	61
***Potato: Plain**	1	250	2	7
With Bacon and Cheese	1	570	30	47
With Broccoli and Cheese	1	500	25	45
With Cheese	1	590	34	51
With Chili and Cheese	1	510	20	35
With Sour Cream and Chives	1	460	24	47
Potato Salad	1	110	9	74
Taco Salad	1	390	18	42
***Three Bean Salad**	1	60	0	0
***White Bun, Hamburger**	1	140	2	13

■ **WHITE CASTLE**
Fat Range = 21% to 61%
Average Fat = 36%

FOOD	MEASURE OR QUANTITY	CALORIES	FAT GRAMS	% FAT
Cheeseburger	1	260	10	35
Chicken Sandwich	1	264	9	31
***Fish Sandwich**	1	230	6	23
French Fries	1	300	14	42
Hamburger	1	234	9	35
Onion Chips	1	330	17	46
Onion Rings	1	245	13	48
Sausage and Egg Sandwich	1	325	22	61

11. FATS AND OILS

■ BUTTER
Fat Range = 94% to 100% Fat
Average Fat = 98%

FOOD	MEASURE OR QUANTITY	CALORIES	FAT GRAMS	% FAT
Butter, Clarified	4 oz	910	100	99
Butter Oil	1 cup	1830	204	100
Butter Oil	1 T	114	12	95
Butter, Salted Regular	1 t	36	4	100
Butter, Salted Regular	1 pat	36	4	100
Butter, Salted Regular	1 T	115	12	94
Butter, Salted Regular	1 stick	815	90	99
Butter, Salted Regular	1 cup	1645	183	100
Butter, Salted Whipped	1 t	27	3	100
Butter, Salted Whipped	1 T	72	8	100
Butter, Salted Whipped	4 oz	540	60	100
Butter, Salted Whipped	1 cup	1080	120	100
Butter, Unsalted Regular	1 cup	1645	183	100
Butter, Unsalted Regular	1 stick	815	90	99
Butter, Unsalted Regular	1 T	115	12	94
Butter, Unsalted Regular	1 t	36	4	100
Butter, Unsalted Whipped	1 cup	1080	120	100
Butter, Unsalted Whipped	4 oz	540	60	100
Butter, Unsalted Whipped	1 T	72	8	100
Butter, Unsalted Whipped	1 t	36	4	100

■ BUTTER SUBSTITUTES
Fat Range = 0% to 100% Fat
Average Fat = 50%

FOOD	MEASURE OR QUANTITY	CALORIES	FAT GRAMS	% FAT
*Butter-Buds	2 t	12	0	0
"I Can't Believe It's Not Butter"[1] (Mrs. Filbert's)	1 T	90	10	100
Molly McButter:				
*Butter Flavor	2 t	16	0	0
*Sour Cream & Butter	2 t	16	0	0
Shedd's:				
Butter Blend[1]	1 T	90	10	100
Country Crock[1]	1 T	50	5	90

[1]Contains saturated fat.

■ FATS AND SHORTENINGS
Fat Range = 100% Fat
Average Fat = 100%

FOOD	MEASURE OR QUANTITY	CALORIES	FAT GRAMS	% FAT
Beef Tallow (Lard)	1 T	117	13	100
Beef Tallow (Lard)	1 cup	1850	205	100
Chicken Fat	1 T	117	13	100
Crisco[1]	1 T	117	13	100
Duck Fat	1 T	117	13	100
Goose Fat	1 T	117	13	100
Lard	1 T	117	13	100
Lard	1 cup	1850	205	100
Mutton Tallow	1 T	117	13	100
Shortening:				
Lard	1 cup	1850	205	100
Lard	1 T	117	13	100
Vegetable	1 cup	1850	205	100
Vegetable	1 T	117	13	100
Turkey Fat	1 T	117	13	100

■ MARGARINE
Fat Range = 90% to 100% Fat
Average Fat = 98%

FOOD	MEASURE OR QUANTITY	CALORIES	FAT GRAMS	% FAT
Blue Bonnet:				
Imitation Diet	1 T	50	5	90
Regular	1 T	100	11	99
Soft	1 T	90	10	100
Whipped	1 T	70	7	90
Corn	1 T	50	5	90
Corn	1 t	20	2	90
Country Crock (Shedd's)	1 T	70	7	90
Country Morning Blend, Light	1 t	20	2	90
Fleischmann's:				
Imitation Diet	1 T	50	5	90
Regular	1 T	100	11	99
Unsalted	1 T	100	11	99
Whipped	1 T	70	7	90
Hain	1 T	100	11	99
Imperial:				
Regular	1 T	100	11	99
Soft	1 T	100	11	99
Whipped	1 T	50	5	90
Kraft	1 T	50	5	90
Mazola:				
Imitation Diet	1 T	50	5	90

[1]Monosaturated fat.

FOOD	MEASURE OR QUANTITY	CALORIES	FAT GRAMS	% FAT
Regular	1 T	100	11	99
Unsalted	1 T	100	11	99
Mother's Unsalted	1 T	100	11	99
Mrs. Filbert's	1 T	100	11	99
Nucoa	1 T	100	11	99
Nucoa	1 cup	1420	158	100
Nucoa, Soft	1 T	100	11	99
Parkay:				
Diet	1 T	50	5	90
Regular	1 T	60	5	75
Promise, Extra Light	1 T	55	6	98
Store Brand	1 T	100	11	99
Weight Watchers:				
Diet	1 T	50	5	90
Light Spread	1 T	55	6	98
Reduced Calorie	1 T	55	6	98

■ MAYONNAISE, REAL AND IMITATION

Fat Range = 75% to 100% Fat
Average Fat = 93%

FOOD	MEASURE OR QUANTITY	CALORIES	FAT GRAMS	% FAT
Best Foods	1 T	100	11	99
Best Foods	1 cup	1570	175	100
Borden's	1 T	100	11	99
Hellmann's:				
Light	1 T	50	5	90
Light	1 cup	760	78	92
Real	1 T	100	11	99
Real	1 cup	1570	175	100
Sandwich Spread	1 T	60	5	75
Kraft:				
Light Reduced Calorie	1 T	45	5	100
Miracle Whip (Kraft):				
Light	1 T	44	4	82
Regular	1 T	70	7	90
Regular	1 T	100	11	99
Mrs. Filbert's:				
Regular	1 T	100	11	99
Imitation	1 T	40	4	90
Soybean Imitation (Store Brand)	1 T	36	3	75
Weight Watchers	1 T	40	4	90

■ OIL SPRAYS
Fat Range = 0% Fat
Average Fat = 0%

FOOD	MEASURE OR QUANTITY	CALORIES	FAT GRAMS	% FAT
*Mazola	2-second spray	4	0	0
*Pam	2-second spray	4	0	0
*Weight Watchers	2-second spray	4	0	0

■ OILS
Fat Range = 64% to 100% Fat
Average Fat = 97%

FOOD	MEASURE OR QUANTITY	CALORIES	FAT GRAMS	% FAT
Blue Bonnet Light Tasty Vegetable[1]	1 T	60	7	105
Blue Bonnet Vegetable[1]	1 t	80	8	90
Coconut[2]	1 T	130	14	97
Cod Liver (Hain)[3]	1 T	135	15	100
Cod Liver[3]	1 T	135	15	100
Cod Liver, Cherry (Hain)[3]	1 T	135	15	100
Cod Liver, Lemon (Hain)[3]	1 T	210	15	64
Cod Liver, Mint (Hain)[3]	1 T	135	15	100
Corn[1]	1 t	50	5	90
Corn[1]	1 cup	1930	215	100
Corn[1]	1 T	130	14	97
Corn (Crisco)[1]	1 T	130	14	97
Cottonseed[1]	1 T	130	14	97
Cottonseed[1]	1 cup	1930	215	100
Olive[3]	1 cup	1930	214	100
Olive[3]	1 T	130	14	97
Olive (Bertolli)[3]	1 T	130	14	97
Palm[2]	1 T	130	14	97
Peanut[3]	1 cup	1930	215	100
Peanut (Planter's)[3]	1 T	130	14	97
Peanut[3]	1 T	130	14	97
Popcorn (Orville Redenbacher's)[1]	1 T	130	14	97
Popcorn (Planters)[1]	1 T	130	14	97
Rapeseed[1]	1 cup	1930	215	100
Rapeseed[1]	1 T	135	15	100
Rice Bran[1]	1 T	130	14	97

Note: Hydrogenation increases the level of saturation.
[1]Polyunsaturated fat.
[2]Saturated fat.
[3]Monosaturated fat.

FOOD	MEASURE OR QUANTITY	CALORIES	FAT GRAMS	% FAT
Rice Bran[1]	1 cup	1930	215	100
Safflower[1]	1 cup	1930	215	100
Safflower[1]	1 T	130	14	97
Sesame[1]	1 cup	1930	215	100
Sesame[1]	1 T	130	14	97
Soybean[1]	1 t	50	5	90
Soybean[1]	1 cup	1930	215	100
Soybean[1]	1 T	130	14	97
Sunflower[1]	1 cup	1930	215	100
Sunflower[1]	1 T	130	14	97
Walnut[2]	1 T	130	14	97
Wheat Germ[1]	1 T	130	14	97

12. FISH AND SEAFOOD

■ **FISH**
Fat Range = 0% to 70%
Average Fat = 30%

FOOD	MEASURE OR QUANTITY	CALORIES	FAT GRAMS	% FAT
Abalone, Fried	3 oz	160	6	34
Anchovies in Olive Oil	5	40	2	45
Bass, Fried	3-½ oz	200	9	40
*Bass, Black, Raw	4 oz	100	1	9
*Bass, White, Raw	3-½ oz	100	2	18
Blue Fish, Baked	4 oz	140	5	32
Burbot:				
Fried	3-½ oz	170	6	32
*Raw	3-½ oz	80	1	11
Carp, Raw	3-½ oz	115	4	31
*Catfish, Raw	3-½ oz	100	3	27
Caviar, Sturgeon	1 T	40	2	45
Caviar, Sturgeon	1 oz	74	4	49
*Clams, Cherrystones, Steamed	4	60	1	15
*Clams, Littlenecks, Steamed	5	60	1	15
*Cod, Broiled	3-½ oz	170	5	26
Crab:				
Deviled	3-½ oz	190	9	43
*Steamed	1 cup	120	2	15
*Crab, Blue, Steamed	6-½ oz	125	3	22

Note: Hydrogenation increases the level of saturation.
[1]Polyunsaturated fat.
[2]Monosaturated fat.

FOOD	MEASURE OR QUANTITY	CALORIES	FAT GRAMS	% FAT
*Crab, King, Steamed	7-½ oz	180	5	25
*Crayfish, Freshwater,				
Steamed	3-½ oz	70	1	13
*Croaker, Atlantic, Baked	3-½ oz	130	3	21
Eel, American, Boiled	3-½ oz	230	18	70
Flounder:				
Fried	3-½ oz	200	8	36
*Raw	3-½ oz	80	1	11
Haddock:				
Fried	3-½ oz	160	6	34
*Raw	3-½ oz	80	1	11
Halibut:				
Fried	3-½ oz	170	7	37
*Raw	3-½ oz	100	1	9
Herring in Tomato Sauce	1 piece	100	6	54
*Lobster, Steamed	3-½ oz	100	2	18
*Lobster Tail, Steamed	6 oz	175	1	5
Mackerel, Fried	3-½ oz	240	16	60
*Mussels, Steamed	3-½ oz	70	1	13
*Octopus, Steamed	3-½ oz	70	1	13
Oysters:				
Fried	1 oz	70	4	51
*Raw	3 pieces	20	0	0
Pompano, Broiled	3-½ oz	160	9	51
*Perch, Raw	3-½ oz	120	4	30
*Pike, Raw	3-½ oz	90	1	10
*Rockfish, Steamed	3-½ oz	100	3	27
Sablefish, Raw	3-½ oz	200	15	68
Salmon, Broiled with Butter	3-½ oz	190	7	33
Sardines:				
In Oil	3-½ oz	200	11	50
In Tomato Sauce	3-½ oz	200	12	54
*Scallops, Sea or Bay, Steamed	3-½ oz	110	1	8
Scallops, Sea, Fried	3-½ oz	200	8	36
Scallops, Sea, Fried	1 piece	20	1	45
Shad:				
Baked	3-½ oz	200	11	50
Raw	3-½ oz	170	10	53
Shrimp:				
Boiled:				
*Large	10	70	1	13
*Medium	10	40	0	0
*Small	10	30	0	0
Fried	3-½ oz	230	11	43
*Snapper, Baked	3-½ oz	100	1	9
Sole:				
Fried	3-½ oz	200	8	36
*Raw	3-½ oz	80	1	11
Swordfish:				
*Broiled	3-½ oz	180	6	30
*Raw	3-½ oz	120	4	30
Tile Fish:				
*Baked	3-½ oz	140	4	26
*Raw	3-½ oz	80	1	11
*Trout, Raw	3-½ oz	100	2	18

FOOD	MEASURE OR QUANTITY	CALORIES	FAT GRAMS	% FAT
Trout, Lake, Broiled	3-½ oz	170	10	53
Tuna:				
In Oil	3-½ oz	300	21	63
*In Water	3-½ oz	130	1	7
Weakfish:				
Broiled	3-½ oz	200	11	50
Raw	3-½ oz	120	6	45
Whitefish, Smoked	3-½ oz	160	7	39
Yellowtail, Broiled	3-½ oz	140	5	32

■ SEAFOOD COMBINATIONS
Fat Range = 0% to 78%
Average Fat = 44%

FOOD	MEASURE OR QUANTITY	CALORIES	FAT GRAMS	% FAT
Cakes, Fish:				
Regular (Mrs. Paul's)	2 pieces	220	8	33
Thin (Mrs. Paul's)	2 pieces	290	13	40
***Clam Juice** (Borden's)	3 oz	14	0	0
Crabs, Deviled (Mrs. Paul's)	1 piece	170	6	32
Fillet:				
Batter Dipped:				
(Mrs. Paul's)	2 pieces	360	19	48
(Van de Kamp's)	3 oz	180	10	50
Buttered (Mrs. Paul's)	2 pieces	210	13	56
Catch of the Day				
(Van de Kamp's)	5 oz	100	4	36
Crispy Crunch (Mrs. Paul's)	2 pieces	310	16	46
Crunchy Light (Mrs. Paul's)	2 pieces	310	16	46
Crunchy Microwave (Gorton's)	2 pieces	350	26	67
Light Breaded (Mrs. Paul's)	1 piece	290	13	40
Light and Crispy				
(Van de Kamp's)	2 oz	180	15	75
Seasoned (Van de Kamp's)	2 oz	200	10	45
Fish Sticks:				
Breaded (Gorton's)	3 pieces	200	11	50
Crispy Crunch (Mrs. Paul's)	4 pieces	200	10	45
Crunchy Light (Mrs. Paul's)	4 pieces	240	13	49
Crunchy Microwave (Gorton's)	6 pieces	340	22	58
Light and Crispy				
(Van de Kamp's)	4 pieces	270	20	67
Potato Crisp (Gorton's)	4 pieces	260	16	55
Tempura (Gorton's)	3 pieces	200	13	58
(Van de Kamp's)	4 pieces	220	15	61
Flounder:				
Breaded (Van de Kamp's)	1 piece	300	15	45
Crispy Crunch (Mrs. Paul's)	2 pieces	280	15	48
Light Breaded (Mrs. Paul's)	1 piece	320	16	45
Light Recipe (Gorton's)	5 oz	260	11	38
Gefilte Fish:				
*Broth (Mother's)	1 piece	70	1	13

FOOD	MEASURE OR QUANTITY	CALORIES	FAT GRAMS	% FAT
*Jelled (Mother's)	1 piece	70	1	13
(Rokeach)	1 piece	50	2	36
Haddock:				
Batter Dipped				
(Van de Kamp's)	2 pieces	240	10	38
Breaded (Van de Kamp's)	1 piece	300	20	60
Crispy Crunch (Mrs. Paul's)	2 pieces	280	15	48
Light Breaded (Mrs. Paul's)	1 piece	320	14	39
Light and Crispy				
(Van de Kamp's)	1 piece	180	15	75
Light Recipe (Gorton's)	5 oz	270	12	40
Halibut:				
Batter Dipped (Van de Kamp's)	3 pieces	260	15	52
Breaded (Van de Kamp's)	1 piece	220	10	41
Kabobs, Batter Dipped				
(Van de Kamp's)	1 piece	240	15	56
Lox, Smoked (Store Brand)	4 oz	140	5	32
Nova, Smoked (Store Brand)	4 oz	140	5	32
Nuggets, Light and Crispy				
(Van de Kamp's)	2 oz	130	10	69
*Oysters (Bumble Bee)	4 oz	110	3	25
*Parmesan, Fish (Mrs. Paul's)	1 piece	520	11	19
Perch:				
Batter Dipped (Van de Kamp's)	2 pieces	270	15	50
Light and Crispy				
(Van de Kamp's)	1 piece	170	10	53
Salmon:				
Keta (Bumble Bee)	4 oz	155	6	35
Pink:				
(Bumble Bee)	4 oz	155	7	41
(Del Monte)	4 oz	160	7	39
Red (Del Monte)	4 oz	180	9	45
Red Sockeye (Bumble Bee)	4 oz	188	10	48
Smoked (Store Brand)	4 oz	140	5	32
Tomato Sauce (Del Monte)	4 oz	160	7	39
Sardines, Oil:				
(Durkee)	4 oz	280	20	64
(King David)	4 oz	300	23	69
*Scallops, Fried (Mrs. Paul's)	3-½ oz	210	7	30
Shrimp, Fried (Mrs. Paul's)	3 oz	190	10	47
Sole:				
Batter Dipped (Van de Kamp's)	2 pieces	250	15	54
Breaded (Van de Kamp's)	1 piece	300	15	45
Light Breaded (Mrs. Paul's)	1 piece	280	13	42
Light Recipe (Gorton's)	5 oz	260	11	38
Tuna, Chunk Light:				
Oil:				
(Bumble Bee)	4 oz	265	19	65
(Star Kist)	2 oz	170	13	69
Water:				
*(Bumble Bee)	4 oz	117	1	8
*(Star Kist)	2 oz	60	1	15
*Tuna, Dietetic (Star Kist)	2 oz	70	1	13
Tuna, Light Solid:				
Oil (Star Kist)	2 oz	150	13	78
*Water (Star Kist)	2 oz	60	1	15

FOOD	MEASURE OR QUANTITY	CALORIES	FAT GRAMS	% FAT
Tuna, Solid White:				
Oil (Bumble Bee)	4 oz	285	20	63
*Water (Bumble Bee)	4 oz	130	1	7
Tuna, White Chunk, Oil				
(Star Kist)	2 oz	140	10	64
Tuna, White Solid, Oil (Star Kist)	2 oz	140	10	64
Whitefish and Pike:				
*Jelled (Mother's)	1 piece	60	1	15
*(Rokeach)	1 piece	60	1	15

13. FROZEN DESSERTS

■ **FROZEN PUDDING POPS**
Fat Range = 20% to 55%
Average Fat = 31%

FOOD	MEASURE OR QUANTITY	CALORIES	FAT GRAMS	% FAT
***All Flavors, Pudding Stix**				
(Good Humor)	1	90	2	20
Chocolate:				
*(Jell-O)	1	75	2	24
*and Vanilla (Jell-O)	1	70	2	26
With Chocolate Coating (Jell-O)	1	130	8	55
***Chocolate Fudge** (Jell-O)	1	70	2	26
***Chocolate, Milk** (Jell-O)	1	70	2	26
***Chocolate Swirl** (Jell-O)	1	70	2	26
Vanilla:				
*(Jell-O)	1	70	2	26
With Chocolate Coating (Jell-O)	1	130	7	48

■ **FROZEN YOGURT**
Fat Range = 8% to 55%
Average Fat = 23%

FOOD	MEASURE OR QUANTITY	CALORIES	FAT GRAMS	% FAT
***All Flavors** (TCBY)	4 oz	110	0	0
***Black Cherry** (Sealtest)	4 oz	100	2	18

FOOD	MEASURE OR QUANTITY	CALORIES	FAT GRAMS	% FAT
Blueberry:				
Danny (Dannon)	1 cup	210	2	9
Danny-Yo (Dannon)	3.5 oz	120	1	8
Boysenberry Carob:				
Danny (Dannon)	1 bar	140	8	51
Chocolate:				
Danny (Dannon)	1 bar	60	1	15
Danny (Dannon)	1 cup	190	3	14
Chocolate, Diet (Tuscan)	1 bar	140	9	58
Chocolate with Chocolate Coating (Dannon)	1 bar	130	8	55
*Peach (Sealtest)	4 oz	100	2	18
Pina Colada:				
Danny (Dannon)	1 bar	70	1	13
Danny (Dannon)	1 cup	230	4	16
Raspberry:				
Danny (Dannon)	1 cup	210	2	9
Danny-Yo (Dannon)	3.5 oz	110	1	8
*Raspberry, Red (Sealtest)	4 oz	100	2	18
Raspberry with Chocolate Coating (Dannon)	1 bar	130	7	48
Strawberry:				
Danny (Dannon)	1 cup	210	2	9
Danny-Yo (Dannon)	3.5 oz	110	2	16
*(Sealtest)	4 oz	100	2	18
Strawberry with Chocolate Coating	1 bar	130	7	48
Vanilla:				
*(Colombo)	4 oz	100	2	18
Danny (Dannon)	1 bar	60	1	15
Danny (Dannon)	1 cup	180	2	10
Danny-Yo (Dannon)	3.5 oz	110	1	8
Vanilla with Chocolate Coating (Dannon)	1 Bar	130	8	55

■ ICE CREAM AND ICE MILK

Fat Range = 8% to 87%
Average Fat = 44%

FOOD	MEASURE OR QUANTITY	CALORIES	FAT GRAMS	% FAT
Bavarian Mint Nuggets (Carnation)	5	160	12	68
Bon Bons (Carnation):				
Chocolate	5	170	12	64
Vanilla	5	160	12	68
*Bubble Crazy (Good Humor)	1	74	1	12
Bubble-O-Bill (Good Humor)	1	150	8	48
Butter Almond (Breyers)	4 fl oz	170	10	53

FOOD	MEASURE OR QUANTITY	CALORIES	FAT GRAMS	% FAT
Butter Pecan:				
(Häagen-Dazs)	4 fl oz	310	24	70
(Lady Borden)	4 fl oz	180	12	60
Carob (Häagen Dazs)	4 fl oz	260	17	59
Cherry Vanilla				
(Häagen Dazs)	4 fl oz	260	17	59
Chip Crunch Bar (Good Humor)	1	200	14	63
Chocolate:				
(Baskin-Robbins)	1 scoop	165	8	44
(Ben & Jerry's)	4 fl oz	290	18	56
(Borden's)	4 fl oz	160	10	56
(Breyers)	4 fl oz	160	8	45
(Häagen Dazs)	4 fl oz	280	17	55
(Steve's Light)	4 fl oz	190	8	38
(Store Brand)	4 fl oz	150	7	42
Chocolate Chip:				
Chocolate (Breyers)	4 fl oz	180	10	50
(Häagen Dazs)	4 fl oz	310	18	52
*Chocolate Cream				
(Weight Watchers)	5 fl oz	120	1	8
Chocolate, Dark Coated Bar				
(Häagen Dazs)	1	360	25	62
Chocolate, Deep (Häagen Dazs)	4 fl oz	330	19	52
Chocolate, Dutch:				
Almond (Borden's)	4 fl oz	160	9	51
(Borden's)	4 fl oz	130	6	42
*(Weight Watchers)	5 fl oz	100	1	9
Chocolate Fudge				
(Baskin-Robbins)	1 scoop	180	9	45
Chocolate Fudge Cake				
(Good Humor)	1	260	16	55
*Chocolate Ice Milk (Borden's)	4 fl oz	110	3	25
Chocolate Malt Bar				
(Good Humor)	1	190	13	62
Chocolate Mint:				
(Baskin-Robbins)	1 scoop	160	9	51
Chocolate (Häagen Dazs)	4 fl oz	300	20	60
*Treat (Weight Watchers)	2 fl oz	60	1	15
Chocolate Mousse				
(Baskin-Robbins)	1 scoop	180	9	45
Chocolate Nuggets (Carnation)	5	180	13	65
Chocolate, Soft (Store Brand)	4 fl oz	180	8	40
Chocolate, Swiss Almond				
(Häagen Dazs)	4 fl oz	250	17	61
*Chocolate Treat (Weight Watchers)	3 fl oz	100	1	9
Coconut Bar (Good Humor)	1	200	14	63
Coffee:				
(Häagen Dazs)	4 fl oz	270	17	57
*(Light 'n Lively)	4 fl oz	100	3	27
(Steve's Light)	4 fl oz	190	8	38
Cookies and Cream:				
(Breyers)	4 fl oz	170	9	48
(Häagen Dazs)	4 fl oz	270	17	57
*(Light 'n Lively)	4 fl oz	120	3	22
Cookie Sandwich (Good Humor)	1	290	11	34

FOOD	MEASURE OR QUANTITY	CALORIES	FAT GRAMS	% FAT
Crunch Bar:				
(Eskimo Pie)	1	170	12	64
Junior (Eskimo Pie)	1	100	8	72
*Double Fudge (Weight Watchers)	2 fl oz	60	1	15
Eclair Bar (Good Humor)	1	180	9	45
Eskimo Pie:				
Chocolate	1	170	12	64
Junior	1	100	7	63
Original	1	140	10	64
Fat Frog (Good Humor)	1	140	7	45
Fudge Nut Fantasy				
(Steve's Light)	4 fl oz	200	8	36
Fudge Toffee Parfait				
(Breyers Light)	4 fl oz	140	5	32
Heart (Good Humor)	1	200	12	54
Heath Bar Crunch				
(Steve's Light)	4 fl oz	210	8	34
Heavenly Hash:				
*Light (Breyers)	4 fl oz	150	5	30
*(Light 'n Lively)	4 fl oz	120	3	22
Jamoca (Baskin-Robbins)	1 scoop	150	8	48
Macadamia Nut (Häagen Dazs)	4 fl oz	260	19	66
Maple Walnut (Häagen Dazs)	4 fl oz	290	19	59
Mocha Chip (Häagen Dazs)	4 fl oz	260	19	66
Mocha Double Nut				
(Häagen Dazs)	4 fl oz	290	20	62
Neapolitan:				
(Breyers)	4 fl oz	150	8	48
*(Light 'n Lively)	4 fl oz	110	3	25
*(Weight Watchers)	5 fl oz	100	1	9
New York Super Fudge				
(Steve's Light)	4 fl oz	200	8	36
*Orange-Vanilla Treat				
(Weight Watchers)	2 fl oz	60	1	15
Oreo Cookies 'n Cream:				
(Häagen Dazs)	4 fl oz	140	8	51
Mint	4 fl oz	160	9	51
Sandwich	1	240	11	41
Stick	1	220	15	61
Vanilla	4 fl oz	160	9	51
Peach, Elberta (Häagen Dazs)	4 fl oz	250	16	58
Peanut Butter Vanilla				
(Häagen Dazs)	4 fl oz	280	20	64
Praline Almond Crunch				
(Breyers Light)	4 fl oz	130	5	35
Pralines and Cream:				
(Baskin-Robbins)	1 scoop	180	8	40
(Häagen Dazs)	4 fl oz	260	16	55
(Light 'n Lively)	4 fl oz	140	5	32
*Raspberry Vanilla & Cream				
(Chiquita)	1	80	1	11
Rocky Road (Baskin-Robbins)	1 scoop	180	7	35
Rum Raisin (Häagen Dazs)	4 fl oz	260	16	55
Strawberry:				
(Baskin-Robbins)	1 scoop	140	6	39
(Borden's)	4 fl oz	120	5	38

FOOD	MEASURE OR QUANTITY	CALORIES	FAT GRAMS	% FAT
(Breyers)	4 fl oz	135	7	47
(Chiquita)	1	80	3	34
(Häagen Dazs)	4 fl oz	270	26	87
(Steve's Light)	4 fl oz	170	6	32
(Store Brand)	4 fl oz	130	5	35
*Strawberry Banana (Chiquita)	1	80	2	22
*Strawberry Ice Milk (Borden's)	4 fl oz	110	3	25
Strawberry Shortcake (Good Humor)	1	186	12	58
Strawberry, Soft	4 fl oz	160	6	34
Sundae (Good Humor)	1	300	11	33
Toasted Almond (Good Humor)	1	190	8	38
Toasted Caramel (Good Humor)	1	170	9	48
Vanilla:				
All Natural (Borden's)	4 fl oz	140	7	45
(Baskin-Robbins)	1 scoop	150	8	48
(Borden's)	4 fl oz	130	7	48
(Breyers)	4 fl oz	150	8	48
(Eskimo Pie)	1	170	12	64
(Eskimo Pie Light)	1 bar	140	9	58
(Good Humor)	1	170	11	58
(Häagen Dazs)	4 fl oz	270	17	57
*(Light 'n Lively)	4 fl oz	100	3	27
(Steve's Light)	4 fl oz	190	8	38
(Store Brand)	4 fl oz	140	7	45
Vanilla Chocolate Chip (Häagen Dazs)	4 fl oz	280	17	55
Vanilla Chocolate Cup (Good Humor)	1	200	9	40
Vanilla, Cool 'n Creamy (Crystal Light)	1	55	2	33
Vanilla, Dark Chocolate Coated Bar (Häagen Dazs)	1	330	23	63
Vanilla, French:				
(Baskin-Robbins)	1 scoop	180	12	60
(Ben & Jerry's)	4 fl oz	270	17	57
(Borden's)	4 fl oz	150	8	48
(Lady Borden's)	4 fl oz	170	9	48
*Vanilla Golden (Weight Watchers)	5 fl oz	100	1	9
Vanilla, Honey (Häagen Dazs)	4 fl oz	250	16	58
*Vanilla Ice Cream Sandwich (Good Humor)	1	170	5	26
*Vanilla Ice Milk (Borden's)	4 fl oz	100	3	27
*(Light 'n Lively)	4 fl oz	110	3	25
*(Weight Watchers)	5 fl oz	100	1	9
Vanilla Milk Chocolate Coated Bar (Häagen Dazs)	1	330	23	63
Vanilla Nuggets (Carnation)	5	170	12	64
Vanilla, Old Fashioned (Eskimo Pie)	1	280	21	68
Vanilla, Original (Eskimo Pie)	1	140	10	64
*Vanilla Raspberry Twirl (Light 'n Lively)	4 fl oz	110	3	25
*Vanilla Sandwich Bar (Weight Watchers)	3 oz	130	2	14

FOOD	MEASURE OR QUANTITY	CALORIES	FAT GRAMS	% FAT
Vanilla Slices (Good Humor)	1	110	6	49
Vanilla, Soft	4 fl oz	170	8	42
Vanilla, Swiss Almond				
(Häagen Dazs)	4 fl oz	340	24	64
Whammy (Good Humor)	1	90	6	60

■ ICE CREAM CONES
Fat Range = 0% to 17%
Average Fat = 8%

FOOD	MEASURE OR QUANTITY	CALORIES	FAT GRAMS	% FAT
***Cone, Chocolate Chip**				
(General Mills)	1	110	2	16
Cone, Sugar:				
*(Comet)	1	40	0	0
*(Disney)	1	53	1	17
***Cone, Vanilla** (General Mills)	1	110	2	16
Cone, Waffle:				
*(Disney)	1	60	1	15
*Specialty (Ice Cream Shop)	1	200	3	14
Cup, Plain:				
*(Disney)	1	18	0	0
*(Keebler)	1	15	0	0
***Cup, Cake** (Comet)	1	20	0	0
***Cup, Chocolate** (Comet)	1	25	0	0

■ ICE CREAM CONES AND ICE CREAM
SUPERMARKET NON-GOURMET BRAND
Fat Range = 42% to 50%
Average Fat = 45%

FOOD	MEASURE OR QUANTITY	CALORIES	FAT GRAMS	% FAT
Chocolate Ice Cream Cone:				
1 Scoop	1	180	10	50
2 Scoops	1	360	20	50
Vanilla Ice Cream Cone:				
1 Scoop	1	170	8	42
2 Scoops	1	320	16	45

■ ICE CREAM SUNDAES

ONE CUP OF NON-GOURMET ICE CREAM + 2 T OF SYRUP + 2 T WHIPPING CREAM
Fat Range = 42% to 44%
Average Fat = 43%

FOOD	MEASURE OR QUANTITY	CALORIES	FAT GRAMS	% FAT
Banana Split with 3 Scoops Ice Cream	1	700	33	42
Butterscotch:				
With Chocolate Ice Cream	1	555	27	44
With Vanilla Ice Cream	1	535	25	42
Hot Fudge:				
With Chocolate Ice Cream	1	560	27	43
With Vanilla Ice Cream	1	540	25	42

■ ICE CREAM TOPPINGS

Fat Range = 0% to 100%
Average Fat = 25%

FOOD	MEASURE OR QUANTITY	CALORIES	FAT GRAMS	% FAT
Butterscotch:				
*(Kraft)	1 T	60	1	15
*(Smucker's)	1 T	70	0	0
Caramel:				
*(Kraft)	1 T	60	0	0
*(Smucker's)	1 T	70	0	0
*Cherry (Smucker's)	1 T	50	0	0
*Cherry, Maraschino	1	10	0	0
Chocolate:				
*(Kraft)	1 T	60	0	0
Magic Shell (Smucker's)	1 T	90	7	70
*(Smucker's)	1 T	65	0	0
Chocolate Fudge:				
(Hershey's)	1 T	50	2	36
*(Smucker's)	1 T	65	0	0
Chocolate Nut, Magic Shell				
(Smucker's)	1 T	100	8	72
Cool Whip:				
Extra Creamy	1 T	18	2	100
Regular	1 T	11	1	82
*Hot Caramel (Smucker's)	1 T	75	2	24
Hot Fudge:				
*(Kraft)	1 T	70	0	0
*(Smucker's)	1 T	75	2	24
Marshmallow:				
*(Kraft)	1 T	90	0	0
*(Smucker's)	1 T	70	0	0
Nut Topping (Planters)	1 oz	180	16	80
*Peanut Butter Magic				
(Smucker's)	1 T	75	1	12

FOOD	MEASURE OR QUANTITY	CALORIES	FAT GRAMS	% FAT
*Pecans In Syrup (Smucker's)	1 T	65	0	0
Pineapple:				
*(Kraft)	1 T	50	0	0
*(Smucker's)	1 T	65	0	0
*Sprinkles, Chocolate	1 T	30	0	0
*Sprinkles, Colored	1 T	30	0	0
Strawberry:				
*(Kraft)	1 T	50	0	0
*(Smucker's)	1 T	60	0	0
*Swiss Milk Fudge (Smucker's)	1 T	75	0	0
Walnuts (Kraft)	1 T	90	5	50
*Walnuts in Syrup (Smucker's)	1 T	65	0	0
Whipping Cream:				
Plain	1 T	45	5	100
Non-Dairy Pressurized	1 T	12	1	75
Pressurized	1 T	9	1	100

■ ICES AND FROZEN FRUIT
Fat Range = 0% to 30%
Average Fat = 2%

FOOD	MEASURE OR QUANTITY	CALORIES	FAT GRAMS	% FAT
Banana:				
*(Chiquita)	1	80	2	22
*Ice Bar (Dole)	1	80	0	0
*Berry Blend (Crystal Light)	1	14	0	0
*Berry Punch (Jell-O)	1	31	0	0
*Blueberry (Dole)	1	90	1	10
*Boysenberry Ice (Häagen Dazs)	4 fl oz	90	0	0
*Casis Fru It Ice (Häagen Dazs)	4 fl oz	130	0	0
Cherry:				
*(Dole)	1	70	0	0
*(FrozFruit)	1	70	0	0
*Italian Ice	6 fl oz	140	0	0
*(Jell-O)	1	32	0	0
*Cherry Cola Kick (Good Humor)	1	106	1	8
*Cherry Fresh Lites (Dole)	1	25	0	0
*Chocolate, Italian Ice	6 fl oz	150	0	0
*Chocolate, Dutch (American Glacée)	4 fl oz	50	0	0
*Fruit Punch Pops (Crystal Light)	1	14	0	0
*Grape (Weight Watchers)	1	35	0	0
*Ice Stripes (Good Humor)	1	40	0	0
*Jumbo Jet (Good Humor)	1	85	0	0
*Lemon Calippo (Good Humor)	1	112	0	0
Lemon:				
*Ice (Häagen Dazs)	4 fl oz	140	0	0
*Italian Ice	6 fl oz	140	0	0
*Sherbet (Borden's)	4 fl oz	110	1	8
*Lime, Ice (Häagen Dazs)	4 fl oz	130	0	0

FOOD	MEASURE OR QUANTITY	CALORIES	FAT GRAMS	% FAT
Orange:				
*Calippo (Good Humor)	1	110	0	0
*Fruit (Dole)	1	70	0	0
*Ice (Häagen Dazs)	4 fl oz	140	0	0
*Sherbet (Borden's)	4 fl oz	110	1	8
Orange Mandarin:				
*(Dole)	1	70	0	0
*Sorbet (Dole)	4 fl oz	110	0	0
*Peach Sorbet (Dole)	4 fl oz	120	0	0
*Pina Colada (Dole)	1	90	3	30
Pineapple:				
*(Dole)	1	70	0	0
*Sorbet (Dole)	4 fl oz	120	0	0
*Pop Ice	1 fl oz	20	0	0
*Pops, Twin (Eskimo Pie)	3 fl oz	70	0	0
*Push-Up Pop (Good Humor)	1	56	1	16
*Rainbow, Italian Ice	6 fl oz	140	0	0
Raspberry:				
*(Dole)	1	70	0	0
*(FrozFruit)	1	70	0	0
*Ice (Häagen Dazs)	4 fl oz	100	0	0
*Sorbet (Dole)	4 fl oz	110	0	0
*(Weight Watchers)	1	35	0	0
*Raspberry Vanilla and Cream				
(Chiquita)	1	80	1	11
*Shark (Good Humor)	1	70	0	0
*Skinny Dip, All Flavors	4 fl oz	40	0	0
Strawberry:				
*(FrozFruit)	1	70	0	0
Fruit Bar:				
*(Chiquita)	1	50	0	0
*(Dole)	1	70	0	0
*(Weight Watchers)	1	35	0	0
*Sorbet (Dole)	4 fl oz	110	0	0
Vanilla:				
*(American Glacée)	4 fl oz	40	0	0
*Italian Ice	6 fl oz	140	0	0
*Watermelon (FrozFruit)	1	70	0	0

■ NON-DAIRY AND FROZEN TOFU
Fat Range = 0% to 56%
Average Fat = 40%

FOOD	MEASURE OR QUANTITY	CALORIES	FAT GRAMS	% FAT
Cappuccino (Tofutti)	4 fl oz	230	12	47
Chocolate:				
Cuties (Tofutti)	4 fl oz	140	5	32
Supreme (Tofutti)	4 fl oz	210	13	56
*Swirl (Tofutti Lite)	4 fl oz	90	0	0

FOOD	MEASURE OR QUANTITY	CALORIES	FAT GRAMS	% FAT
Mocha Mix:				
Almond Fudge, Non-Diary	4 fl oz	150	8	48
Chocolate, Non-Dairy	4 fl oz	160	10	56
Neapolitan, Non-Dairy	4 fl oz	140	7	45
Strawberry, Non-Dairy	4 fl oz	140	7	45
Toasted Almond, Non-Dairy	4 fl oz	150	9	54
Vanilla, Non-Dairy	4 fl oz	140	7	45
Soft Tofutti, Regular, All Flavors	4 fl oz	160	8	45
***Strawberry Swirl** (Tofutti Lite)	4 fl oz	90	0	0
Tofulite, All Flavors (Baracinni)	4 fl oz	170	9	48
Tofu Time, All Flavors	4 fl oz	220	13	53
Vanilla:				
Cuties (Tofutti)	4 fl oz	130	5	35
Love Drops (Tofutti)	4 fl oz	220	12	49
*Swirl (Tofutti Lite)	4 fl oz	90	0	0
(Tofutti)	4 fl oz	200	11	50
Wildberry (Tofutti)	4 fl oz	210	12	51

14. FROZEN DINNERS

■ **FROZEN DINNERS**
Fat Range = 4% to 86%
Average Fat = 34%

FOOD	MEASURE OR QUANTITY	CALORIES	FAT GRAMS	% FAT
***Beef** (Swanson)	1	320	9	25
Beef and Bean Burrito				
(Swanson)	1	700	30	39
***Beef Burgundy** (Light & Elegant)	1	230	4	16
Beef Chimichigas (El Paso)	1	380	23	54
Beef, Chopped:				
(Hungry-Man)	1	620	37	54
(Le Menu)	1	420	24	51
(Swanson)	1	370	18	44
(Weight Watchers)	1	280	17	55
Beef Chop Suey (Stouffer's)	1	340	12	32
Beef Chow Mein:				
(Chun King)	1	290	20	62
*(Van de Kamp's)	1	310	10	29
Beef Enchiladas:				
(El Paso)	1	210	13	56
(Swanson)	1	515	24	42
Beef, Goulash (Hormel)	1	230	12	47

FOOD	MEASURE OR QUANTITY	CALORIES	FAT GRAMS	% FAT
Beef, Gravy (Banquet)	1	344	13	34
***Beef, Julienne** (Light & Elegant)	1	260	7	24
Beef, Oriental:				
*(Budget Gourmet)	1	300	9	27
*(Healthy Choice)	1	290	6	19
*(Lean Cuisine)	1	270	8	27
Beef Patty Sandwich with Cheese (Kid Cuisine)	1	400	19	43
Beef, Pepper Steak				
*(Armour Lite)	1	260	6	21
(Chun King)	1	250	17	61
Beef Pot Pie (Banquet)	1	450	24	48
***Beef Ragout** (Right Choice)	1	300	8	24
Beef, Short Ribs (Stouffer's)	1	280	20	64
Beef, Sirloin with Herb Sauce (Budget Gourmet)	1	310	18	52
Beef Sirloin Tip:				
*(Healthy Choice)	1	290	6	19
(Le Menu)	1	390	18	42
Beef, Sliced:				
*(Hungry-Man)	1	330	8	22
*(Hungry-Man)	1	490	11	20
*With Barbecue Sauce (Banquet)	1	90	2	20
*With Vegetables (Banquet)	1	300	9	27
Beef Stew (Stouffer's)	1	310	16	46
Beef Stroganoff:				
(Armour)	1	320	11	31
(Stouffer's)	1	410	21	46
(Weight Watchers)	1	340	15	40
*With Noodles (Light & Elegant)	1	260	6	21
***Beef Teriyaki** (Light & Elegant)	1	240	3	11
Cheese Canneloni (Lean Cuisine)	1	270	10	33
Cheese Enchiladas (El Paso)	1	250	12	43
Cheese Manicotti (Budget Gourmet)	1	450	25	50
***Cheese Ravioli Slim Selections** (Budget Gourmet)	1	260	7	24
Chicken A La King:				
(Banquet)	1	160	7	39
(Le Menu)	1	320	14	39
(Stouffer's)	1	320	11	31
(Weight Watchers)	1	230	8	31
Chicken A La Orange (Le Menu)	1	320	13	37
Chicken Au Gratin (Budget Gourmet)	1	260	10	35
Chicken, Barbecue:				
*(Armour)	1	280	8	26
Fried (Swanson)	1	520	24	42
*(Light & Elegant)	1	300	6	18
(Swanson)	1	560	30	48
Chicken, Boneless:				
(Hungry-Man)	1	620	37	54
Large (Hungry-Man)	1	670	27	36

FOOD	MEASURE OR QUANTITY	CALORIES	FAT GRAMS	% FAT
Chicken Breast:				
*(Classic Lite)	1	270	9	30
(Swanson)	1	880	49	50
Chicken Breast Fried:				
(Hungry-Man Dark)	1	890	48	49
(Hungry-Man)	1	870	47	49
(Swanson)	1	650	30	42
***Chicken Breast and**				
Mushrooms (Armour Lite)	1	240	5	19
Chicken with Broccoli				
(Light & Elegant)	1	290	11	34
***Chicken Burgundy** (Armour Lite)	1	200	2	9
Chicken Cacciatore:				
*(Armour Lite)	1	250	4	14
*(Banquet)	1	260	5	17
(Budget Gourmet)	1	300	13	39
(Lean Cuisine)	1	280	10	32
Chicken in Cheese Sauce				
(Light & Elegant)	1	290	11	34
Chicken Chimichigas (El Paso)	1	370	21	51
Chicken Chow Mein:				
*(Chun King)	1	230	5	20
*(Classic Lite)	1	220	4	16
*(La Choy)	1	260	4	14
*(Lean Cuisine)	1	250	5	18
(Stouffer's)	1	140	5	32
Chicken Cordon Bleu (Le Menu)	1	460	19	37
Chicken, Creamed (Stouffer's)	6-½ oz	320	24	68
Chicken Divan (Stouffer's)	8-½ oz	350	22	57
Chicken Escalloped (Stouffer's)	5-¾ oz	260	16	55
Chicken Florentine (Le Menu)	1	480	23	43
***Chicken, French** (Banquet)	1	190	4	19
Chicken, Fried:				
Dark (Swanson)	1	600	31	46
(Kid Cuisine)	1	420	22	47
Chicken, Glazed:				
*(Lean Cuisine)	1	270	8	27
*Light (Le Menu)	1	270	6	20
*(Light & Elegant)	1	240	4	15
***Chicken Hawaiian** (Armour)	1	280	5	16
***Chicken, Herb Roasted**				
(Healthy Choice)	1	260	3	10
***Chicken Imperial**				
(Weight Watchers)	1	230	4	16
Chicken, Mandarin:				
*(Budget Gourmet)	1	290	7	22
*Slim Selections				
(Budget Gourmet)	1	300	6	18
Chicken Marsala:				
*Breast (Armour Lite)	1	250	5	18
*(Classic Lite)	1	270	7	23
***Chicken, Mesquite**				
(Healthy Choice)	1	310	2	6
***Chicken Milan** (Armour)	1	320	10	28
Chicken Nuggets (Kid Cuisine)	1	400	19	43
***Chicken Orange** (Lean Cuisine)	1	270	5	17

FOOD	MEASURE OR QUANTITY	CALORIES	FAT GRAMS	% FAT
Chicken, Oriental:				
*(Armour Lite)	1	250	4	14
*(Classic Lite)	1	250	6	22
*(Healthy Choice)	1	220	2	8
Chicken Parmigiana:				
Breast (Le Menu)	1	400	20	45
(Hungry-Man)	1	820	52	57
*(Light & Elegant)	1	260	6	21
***Chicken Pasta Divan**				
(Healthy Choice)	1	310	4	12
Chicken Patty:				
(Weight Watchers)	1	280	15	48
Fried (Weight Watchers)	1	270	15	50
Chicken Pot Pie:				
(Banquet)	1	450	24	48
Hungry-Man (Swanson)	1	700	37	48
(Swanson)	8 oz	420	24	51
Chicken, Sweet and Sour:				
*(Armour Lite)	1	240	2	8
*(Budget Gourmet)	1	350	7	18
*(Classic Lite)	1	250	3	11
*(Healthy Choice)	1	280	2	6
(Le Menu)	1	450	22	44
(Weight Watchers)	1	460	22	43
Chicken Tenderloin:				
*In BBQ Sauce (Right Choice)	1	270	6	20
*With Peanuts (Right Choice)	1	330	10	27
***Chicken Tenders** (Weight Watchers)	1	250	2	7
Chicken Teriyaki (Dinner Classic)	1	340	15	40
***Chicken and Vegetables** (Lean Cuisine)	1	270	7	23
***Chicken and Vermicelli** (Lean Cuisine)	1	270	7	23
***Chicken and Walnut** (Chun King)	1	315	10	29
Crab Au Gratin With Asparagus (Gorton's)	1	280	13	42
***Fettucini, Slim Selections** (Budget Gourmet)	1	300	10	30
Fish Au Grautin Fillet:				
*(Mrs. Paul's)	1	290	8	25
*(Weight Watchers)	1	210	6	26
Fish Dijon (Mrs. Paul's)	1	280	15	48
***Fish, Divan** (Lean Cuisine)	1	270	9	30
Fish Florentine (Lean Cuisine)	1	240	9	34
Fish Flounder Fillet (Mrs. Paul's Light)	1	260	11	38
Fish, Flounder Stuffed With Shrimp (Gorton's)	1	250	13	47
Fish, Fried (Weight Watchers)	1	220	12	49
Fish Jardiniere (Lean Cuisine)	1	280	10	32
Fish and Pasta Florentine (Mrs. Paul's)	1	240	9	34
Fish Mornay (Mrs. Paul's)	1	280	14	45

FOOD	MEASURE OR QUANTITY	CALORIES	FAT GRAMS	% FAT
Fish 'n Chips:				
(Hungry-Man)	1	770	73	85
(Swanson)	1	310	16	46
Fish, Scrod Stuffed (Gorton's)	1	260	15	52
Franks and Beans (Swanson)	1	550	20	33
Lasagna:				
(Budget Gourmet)	1	420	20	43
(Hungry-Man)	1	420	20	43
*(Light & Elegant)	1	280	5	16
*Slim Selections				
(Budget Gourmet)	1	300	10	30
(Swanson)	1	420	19	41
With Meat (Hungry-Man)	1	680	24	32
Linguini & Scallops Slim Selections				
(Budget Gourmet)	1	280	11	35
Linguini & Shrimp				
(Budget Gourmet)	1	330	15	41
Macaroni and Cheese:				
(Banquet)	1	230	8	31
(Swanson)	1	380	15	36
Macaroni and Beef (Swanson)	1	370	15	36
Meat Loaf:				
(Banquet)	1	240	15	56
(Swanson)	1	510	26	46
Meatball Stew (Lean Cuisine)	1	250	10	36
Mexican (Hungry-Man)	1	900	42	42
*Noodles and Chicken (Swanson)	1	270	9	30
Omelet:				
Cheese (Swanson)	1	400	32	72
Spanish Style (Swanson)	1	250	18	65
*Pasta and Sauce (Banquet)	1	300	8	24
Pasta Shells and Beef (Budget Gourmet)	1	340	15	40
Pasta with Vegetables and Ham (Lean Cuisine)	1	280	13	42
Pepper Steak (Le Menu)	1	360	13	32
*Pizza, Cheese (Kid Cuisine)	1	240	4	15
*Pot Roast (Right Choice)	1	220	7	29
*Ravioli, Mini, Cheese (Kid Cuisine)	1	250	2	7
Rigatoni (Lean Cuisine)	1	260	10	35
Salisbury Steak:				
(Armour Lite)	1	270	12	40
(Banquet)	1	230	18	70
*(Healthy Choice)	1	300	7	21
(Hungry-Man)	1	710	40	51
Scrambled Eggs and Sausage (Swanson)	1	420	35	75
*Seafood & Herbs (Armour Lite)	1	220	4	16
Seafood Newburg (Budget Gourmet)	1	350	12	31
*Shrimp (Armour Lite)	1	260	6	21
*Shrimp Creole (Healthy Choice)	1	210	1	4
*Shrimp Primavera (Right Choice)	1	240	7	26

FOOD	MEASURE OR QUANTITY	CALORIES	FAT GRAMS	% FAT
Sirloin Enchilada Slim Selections				
(Budget Gourmet)	1	300	15	45
Sirloin, Salisbury:				
(Budget Gourmet)	1	410	22	48
*Slim Selections				
(Budget Gourmet)	1	280	8	26
*Sole Au Gratin (Healthy Choice)	1	310	4	12
Sole Fillet (Mrs. Paul's Light)	1	260	11	38
*Sole Stuffed (Weight Watchers)	1	310	9	26
Spaghetti and Meatballs:				
*(Lean Cuisine)	1	280	7	22
(Swanson)	1	410	14	31
Steak Diane (Armour Lite)	1	260	10	35
Swedish Meatballs (Armour)	1	500	30	54
Swiss Steak (Swanson)	1	350	14	36
Tuna Pot Pie (Banquet)	1	400	18	40
Turkey:				
*American (Banquet)	1	320	9	25
*Extra-Helping (Banquet)	1	720	23	29
*(Hungry-Man)	1	590	18	27
*(Morton)	1	280	5	16
*(Swanson)	1	330	10	27
Turkey Breast:				
*(Healthy Choice)	1	290	5	16
Sliced (Le Menu)	1	470	24	46
Turkey Dijon (Lean Cuisine)	1	280	10	32
*Turkey Glazed Slim Selections				
(Budget Gourmet)	1	270	5	17
*Turkey Parmesan (Classic Lite)	1	240	8	30
Turkey Pot Pie:				
(Banquet)	1	435	23	48
(Hungry-Man)	1	740	41	50
(Stouffer's)	1	540	36	60
(Swanson)	8 oz	250	24	86
(Swanson)	10 oz	530	31	53
Turkey, Sliced				
*(Lean Cuisine)	1	220	5	20
*(Right Choice)	1	320	8	22
Turkey, Stuffed				
(Weight Watchers)	1	270	10	33
Turkey Tetrazzini:				
*(Banquet)	1	270	4	13
*(Morton)	1	280	4	13
*Veal Marsala (Le Menu Light)	1	260	6	21
Veal Parmigiana:				
(Banquet)	1	230	11	43
(Hungry-Man)	1	560	25	40
(Swanson)	1	480	25	47
Yankee Pot Roast:				
*(Healthy Choice)	1	220	1	4
(Le Menu)	1	360	15	38

15. FRUITS

■ FRUITS
Fat Range = 0% to 90%
Average Fat = 0%

FOOD	MEASURE OR QUANTITY	CALORIES	FAT GRAMS	% FAT
*Apple	1	81	0	0
*Apple, Dried	1 cup	160	0	0
*Apple Juice	1 cup	120	0	0
Applesauce:				
*Chunky (Mott's)	6 oz	90	0	0
*(Del Monte)	4 oz	90	0	0
*Lite (Del Monte)	4 oz	50	0	0
*(Mott's)	4 oz	90	0	0
*(Seneca)	4 oz	90	0	0
Applesauce, Cinnamon:				
*(Mott's)	6 oz	110	0	0
*(Tree Top)	4 oz	80	0	0
*Applesauce, Golden Delicious				
(Seneca)	4 oz	90	0	0
*Applesauce, McIntosh (Seneca)	4 oz	90	0	0
Applesauce, Natural:				
*(Mott's)	6 oz	70	0	0
*(Seneca)	4 oz	50	0	0
*(Tree Top)	4 oz	60	0	0
*(Whitehouse)	4 oz	50	0	0
Applesauce, Sweetened:				
*(Store Brand)	1 cup	200	0	0
*(S&W)	4 oz	90	0	0
Applesauce, Unsweetened:				
*(Store Brand)	1 cup	108	0	0
*(S&W)	4 oz	55	0	0
*Apples, Sliced	1 cup	68	0	0
*Apricot	1	16	0	0
Apricot, Canned in Syrup:				
*(Store Brand)	1 cup	224	0	0
*(S&W)	4 oz	100	0	0
*Apricot, Candied (Store Brand)	1 oz	100	0	0
*Apricot, Dried	1 cup	340	0	0
Apricot Halves:				
*(Del Monte)	4 oz	100	0	0
*Lite (Del Monte)	4 oz	60	0	0
*Apricot Nectar	1 cup	148	0	0
*Whole (Del Monte)	4 oz	100	0	0
Avocado	1	334	30	81
Avocado Puree (Store Brand)	1 cup	400	40	90
*Banana, Flakes	1 cup	340	1	3
*Banana, Peeled	1	117	1	8

FOOD	MEASURE OR QUANTITY	CALORIES	FAT GRAMS	% FAT
*Blackberries	1 cup	85	0	0
*Blueberries	1 cup	90	1	10
*Boysenberries	1 cup	80	0	0
*Cantaloupe	1 cup	60	0	0
*Cantaloupe 5″ Diameter	½	100	0	0
*Casaba 5″ Diameter	½	100	0	0
*Cherry, Candied	1	12	0	0
*Cherries, Dark Sweet (Del Monte)	4 oz	90	0	0
Cherries, Frozen:				
*Sweetened	1 cup	200	0	0
*Unsweetened	1 cup	100	0	0
*Cherries in Syrup	1 cup	240	0	0
*Cherry, Maraschino	1	10	0	0
*Cherry, Maraschino	1 oz	33	0	0
*Cherries, Pitted	1 cup	80	0	0
*Cherries, Sweet	10	50	0	0
*Cherries, Sweet	1 cup	128	0	0
*Cranberries	1 cup	50	0	0
*Cranberries, Fresh (Ocean Spray)	2 oz	25	0	0
*Cranberries (Ocean Spray)	4 oz	50	0	0
*Cranberry Sauce	1 cup	432	0	0
*Cranberry Sauce, Jellied (Ocean Spray)	2 oz	90	0	0
*Cranberry Sauce (S&W)	2 oz	90	0	0
*Cranberry, Whole Berry (Ocean Spray)	2 oz	90	0	0
*Dates, Chopped	1 cup	500	1	2
*Dates, Dried	1 cup	549	1	2
*Dates, Dried	1	24	0	0
*Dates, Pitted (Dromedary)	5	100	0	0
*Figs	1	40	0	0
*Figs, Dried	1 cup	544	0	0
*Figs, in Syrup	1 cup	244	0	0
*Figs (S&W)	4 oz	100	0	0
*Fruit Cocktail in Heavy Syrup (S&W)	4 oz	90	0	0
*Fruit Cocktail in Syrup	1 cup	196	0	0
*Fruit Cocktail in Water	1 cup	84	0	0
*Fruit Cocktail Lite Syrup (S&W)	4 oz	60	0	0
*Fruit Cocktail Natural (S&W)	4 oz	90	0	0
*Gooseberries	1 cup	64	0	0
*Grapefruit	1	80	0	0
*Grapefruit, Candied	1 oz	90	0	0
*Grapefruit in Syrup (Store Brand)	1 cup	160	0	0
Grapefruit Sections:				
*Lite Syrup (S&W)	4 oz	80	0	0
*(S&W)	4 oz	40	0	0
*Grapefruit 4″ Diameter	½	55	0	0
*Grapes	10	40	0	0
*Grapes, American	1 cup	60	0	0
*Grapes, European	1 cup	112	0	0
*Grapes, in Syrup (S&W)	4 oz	100	0	0

FOOD	MEASURE OR QUANTITY	CALORIES	FAT GRAMS	% FAT
*Grapes (S&W)	4 oz	100	0	0
*Guava	1	48	0	0
*Honey Dew Melon	1 cup	68	0	0
*Honey Dew 5″ Round	½	100	0	0
*Kiwi	1	48	0	0
*Kumquat (Raw)	1	16	0	0
*Lemon (Raw)	1	52	0	0
*Lychees (Raw)	1	8	0	0
*Mango (Raw)	1 cup	144	0	0
*Melon Balls	1	56	0	0
*Mixed Fruit (S&W)	4 oz	90	0	0
*Nectarine	1	68	0	0
*Orange	1	64	0	0
Orange, Mandarin:				
*Heavy Syrup (S&W)	4 oz	60	0	0
*Lite Syrup (S&W)	4 oz	70	0	0
*Orange Peel, Candied	1 oz	90	0	0
*Papaya	1 cup	60	0	0
*Passion Fruit	1 cup	144	0	0
*Peach	1	40	0	0
*Peaches, Dried	1 cup	221	1	4
*Peaches, Dried (Store Brand)	2 oz	140	0	0
Peaches, Halves:				
*(Del Monte)	4 oz	80	0	0
*(S&W)	4 oz	100	0	0
*Peaches Heavy Syrup (S&W)	4 oz	100	0	0
*Peaches in Syrup	1 cup	212	0	0
Peaches Lite Syrup:				
*(Del Monte)	4 oz	50	0	0
*(S&W)	4 oz	50	0	0
*Peach Nectar	1 cup	144	0	0
*Peaches, Sliced	1 cup	80	0	0
*Pear	1	104	0	0
*Pears D'Anjou	1	128	0	0
*Pears (Del Monte)	4 oz	90	0	0
*Pears, Dried (Del Monte)	4 oz	240	2	8
*Pears in Heavy Syrup (S&W)	4 oz	100	0	0
*Pears in Syrup	1 cup	200	0	0
*Persimmon	1	132	0	0
*Pineapple	1 cup	89	1	10
*Pineapple, Candied				
(Store Brand)	1 oz	180	0	0
Pineapple Chunks:				
*Del Monte	4 oz	70	0	0
*Frozen (Store Brand)	4 oz	100	0	0
*In Syrup (Del Monte)	4 oz	90	0	0
*Pineapple, Hawaiian, Sliced				
(S&W)	2	90	0	0
*Pineapple in Juice (Dole)	4 oz	70	0	0
*Pineapple in Syrup	1 cup	136	0	0
*Pineapple in Syrup (Dole)	4 oz	95	0	0
*Pineapple Pieces in Syrup				
(Store Brand)	1 cup	200	0	0
*Pineapple Spears (Del Monte)	2	50	0	0
*Plantain	1	204	0	0

FOOD	MEASURE OR QUANTITY	CALORIES	FAT GRAMS	% FAT
*Plums	1	36	0	0
*Plums, in Syrup	1 cup	262	2	7
*Pomegranate	1	108	0	0
*Prickly Pear	1	40	0	0
*Prunes, Cooked and Juice	1 cup	250	1	4
*Prunes, Dried	1 cup	244	0	0
*Prunes in Sugar	1 cup	324	0	0
*Prunes Moist (Del Monte)	2 oz	120	0	0
*Prunes, Uncooked	10	160	0	0
*Raisins	1 cup	480	0	0
*Raisins (Del Monte)	3 oz	260	0	0
*Raisins (Store Brand)	1 cup	480	0	0
*Raspberries (Raw)	1 cup	60	0	0
*Raspberries, Sweetened	1 cup	90	0	0
*Raspberry Halves, Frozen (Bird's Eye)	5 oz	90	0	0
*Rhubarb	1 cup	50	0	0
*Rhubarb in Syrup	1 cup	100	0	0
*Roselle	1 cup	28	0	0
*Strawberries	1 cup	45	0	0
*Strawberries	1 pt	100	0	0
*Strawberries	1 lb	140	0	0
Strawberry Halves:				
*(Bird's Eye)	5 oz	100	0	0
*In Syrup (Bird's Eye)	5 oz	120	0	0
*Strawberries in Syrup (Quick Thaw)	5 oz	120	0	0
*Strawberries in Lite Syrup (Quick Thaw)	5 oz	60	0	0
*Strawberries, Sliced	1 cup	90	0	0
*Strawberries, Whole in Syrup (Bird's Eye)	4 oz	60	0	0
*Tangerine	1	40	0	0
*Watermelon	1 cup	52	0	0
*Watermelon Wedge 10″ Diameter × 1″ thick	1	150	1	6

■ FRUIT SNACKS

Fat Range = 0% to 20%
Average Fat = 5%

FOOD	MEASURE OR QUANTITY	CALORIES	FAT GRAMS	% FAT
*Apricots, Candied	1 oz	100	0	0
*Berry Bears (Fruit Corners)	1 pkg	100	1	9
*Cherries	10	110	0	0
*Dinosaurs (Sunkist)	1 pkg	100	1	9
*Figs	1 oz	85	0	0
*Fruit Bars (General Foods)	1	90	2	20
Fruit Roll-Ups:				
*(General Foods)	1	50	1	18
*(Sunkist)	1	50	0	0

FOOD	MEASURE OR QUANTITY	CALORIES	FAT GRAMS	% FAT
*Fun Fruits, All Types (Sunkist)	1 oz	105	1	9
*Ginger Root	1 oz	100	0	0
*Grapefruit Peel	1 oz	90	0	0
*Lemon Peel	1 oz	90	0	0
*Letters (Sunkist)	1 pkg	100	1	9
*Numbers (Sunkist)	1 pkg	100	1	9
*Orange Peel	1 oz	90	0	0
*Pear	1 oz	85	0	0
*Pineapple	1 oz	90	0	0
*Shark Bites (Fruit Corners)	1 pkg	100	1	9
*Space Shapes (Sunkist)	1 pkg	100	1	9
*Thunder Jets (Fruit Corners)	1 pkg	100	1	9

16. GRAVIES AND SAUCES

■ GRAVIES
Fat Range - 0% to 68% Fat
Average Fat = 28%

FOOD	MEASURE OR QUANTITY	CALORIES	FAT GRAMS	% FAT
Au Jus:				
*(Durkee)	1 cup	60	0	0
*(Franco-American)	2 fl oz	5	0	0
*(R. T. French)	2 fl oz	8	0	0
*(Store Brand)	1 cup	20	0	0
Beef Gravy:				
(Franco-American)	2 fl oz	25	1	36
(Store Brand)	1 cup	125	5	36
Brown Gravy:				
*(Durkee)	1 cup	60	0	0
*(Heinz)	2 fl oz	30	1	30
*(McCormick)	¼ pkg	22	0	0
*(Pillsbury)	2 fl oz	15	0	0
(R. T. French)	2 fl oz	20	1	45
*(Store Brand)	1 cup	9	0	0
*(Weight Watchers)	2 fl oz	8	0	0
Brown Gravy with Cheese				
(Durkee)	1 cup	316	17	48
Brown Gravy with Mushrooms:				
*(Durkee)	1 cup	60	0	0
*(Weight Watchers)	2 fl oz	12	0	0
Brown Gravy with Onions				
*(Durkee)	1 cup	70	1	13

FOOD	MEASURE OR QUANTITY	CALORIES	FAT GRAMS	% FAT
(Franco-American)	2 fl oz	25	1	36
*(Weight Watchers)	2 fl oz	13	0	0
Chicken Gravy:				
*(Durkee)	1 cup	90	1	10
(Franco-American)	2 fl oz	50	4	72
(Heinz)	2 fl oz	40	3	68
*(McCormick)	¼ pkg	20	0	0
(Pillsbury)	2 fl oz	25	1	36
(R. T. French)	2 fl oz	25	1	36
*(Store Brand)	1 cup	80	2	22
*(Weight Watchers)	2 fl oz	10	0	0
Chicken Gravy, Creamy				
(Durkee)	1 cup	160	9	51
Chicken Gravy, Giblets				
(Franco-American)	2 fl oz	25	1	36
Homestyle Gravy:				
*(Pillsbury)	2 fl oz	15	0	0
(R. T. French)	2 fl oz	25	1	36
Mushroom Gravy:				
*(Durkee)	1 cup	60	1	15
*(Heinz)	2 fl oz	30	1	30
(R. T. French)	2 fl oz	20	1	45
*(Store Brand)	1 cup	70	1	13
Onion Gravy:				
*(Durkee)	1 cup	84	1	11
*(Heinz)	2 fl oz	35	1	26
*(McCormick)	¼ pkg	18	0	0
(R. T. French)	2 fl oz	25	1	36
*(Store Brand)	1 cup	80	1	11
Pork Gravy:				
*(Durkee)	1 cup	70	0	0
(Franco-American)	2 fl oz	40	3	68
(Heinz)	2 fl oz	30	2	60
(R. T. French)	2 fl oz	20	1	45
*(Store Brand)	1 cup	80	2	22
Sloppy Joe Barbecue Sauce:				
With Beef (Libby's)	⅓ cup	110	7	57
With Pork (Libby's)	⅓ cup	120	8	60
*Swiss Steak Gravy (Durkee)	1 cup	40	0	0
Turkey Gravy:				
*(Durkee)	1 cup	90	0	0
(Franco-American)	2 fl oz	30	2	60
(Heinz)	2 fl oz	40	3	68
(R. T. French)	2 fl oz	25	1	36
*(Store Brand)	1 cup	80	2	22

■ SAUCES
Fat Range = 0% to 90% Fat
Average Fat = 21%

FOOD	MEASURE OR QUANTITY	CALORIES	FAT GRAMS	% FAT
*A-1, Steak (Heublein)	1 T	14	0	0
Barbecue:				
*(French's Cattlemen's)	1 T	25	0	0
*Barbecue (Kraft)	2 T	40	1	22
*Barbecue, Garlic (Kraft)	2 T	40	0	0
Barbecue, Hickory Smoke:				
*(Heinz)	1 T	20	0	0
*(Kraft)	2 T	50	1	18
*(Open Pit)	2 T	50	0	0
Barbecue, Hot:				
*(Heinz)	1 T	20	0	0
*Hickory Smoke (Kraft)	2 T	40	1	22
*(Kraft)	2 T	40	1	22
*Zesty (Hunt's)	1 T	25	0	0
*Barbecue, Italian (Kraft)	2 T	45	1	20
*Barbecue, Kansas City (Kraft)	2 T	45	1	20
*Barbecue, Mesquite (Kraft)	2 T	45	1	20
*Barbecue, Mushroom (Heinz)	1 T	20	0	0
*Barbecue, Natural Hickory				
(Hunt's)	1 T	25	0	0
*Barbecue, Natural Original				
(Hunt's)	1 T	20	0	0
Barbecue, Onion:				
*(Heinz)	1 T	20	0	0
*(Kraft)	2 T	50	1	18
*Barbecue, Smoky				
(French's Cattlemen's)	1 T	25	0	0
*Barbecue, Thick 'n Tangy				
(Open Pit)	1 T	25	0	0
Barbecue, Thick 'n Spicy:				
*Chunky (Kraft)	2 T	50	1	18
*Hickory Smoked (Kraft)	2 T	50	1	18
*Honey (Kraft)	2 T	60	1	15
*Kansas City (Kraft)	2 T	60	1	15
*Original (Kraft)	2 T	50	1	18
Bechamel (Campbell's)	2 fl oz	60	5	75
Catsup, Tomato:				
*(Campbell's)	1 T	17	0	0
*(Del Monte)	2 fl oz	60	0	0
*(Heinz)	1 T	18	0	0
*(Hunt's)	1 T	16	0	0
*Lite (Heinz)	1 T	8	0	0
Cheese:				
(Del Monte)	2 fl oz	80	4	45
(Durkee)	1 cup	316	17	48
Chili:				
*(Del Monte)	2 fl oz	70	0	0
(Heinz)	1 T	18	1	50
Clam:				
Red (Store Brand)	4 fl oz	80	3	34
White (Store Brand)	4 fl oz	130	10	69

FOOD	MEASURE OR QUANTITY	CALORIES	FAT GRAMS	% FAT
Cocktail, Seafood:				
*(Del Monte)	2 fl oz	70	0	0
*(Heinz)	1 T	20	0	0
Curry (Store Brand)	4 fl oz	90	5	50
Enchilada:				
*Green Chili				
(Old El Paso)	2 fl oz	17	0	0
Hot:				
*(Del Monte)	4 fl oz	45	0	0
(Old El Paso)	2 fl oz	27	1	33
Mild:				
*(Del Monte)	4 fl oz	45	0	0
(Old El Paso)	2 fl oz	25	1	36
Garlic (Catelli)	5 fl oz	100	5	45
*_Heinz 57_	1 T	15	0	0
Hollandaise (French's)	3 T	45	4	80
Horseradish (Sauceworks)	1 T	54	5	83
Marinara:				
*(Catelli)	5 fl oz	60	1	15
(Ragu)	4 fl oz	90	4	40
*Meat Marinade, Mix (Durkee)	4 fl oz	47	1	19
Meat (Catelli)	5 fl oz	140	9	58
Mushroom (Catelli)	5 fl oz	90	4	40
Newburg and Sherry (Snow's)	1/3 cup	120	8	60
Pizza:				
Cheese (Contadina)	2 fl oz	40	2	45
Chunky Style (Ragu)	3 T	45	2	40
Original, Quick & Easy				
(Contadina)	2 fl oz	40	2	45
Pepperoni:				
*(Contadina)	2 fl oz	25	0	0
(Ragu)	3 T	50	3	54
*Pronto (Catelli)	2 T	20	0	0
Sausage and Mushroom (Ragu)	3 T	40	2	45
*Tomato (Contadina)	2 fl oz	25	0	0
Traditional (Ragu)	3 T	40	2	45
Salsa:				
*Burrito (Del Monte)	2 fl oz	20	0	0
*Chili, Green, Mild (Del Monte)	2 fl oz	20	0	0
*Picante, Hot (Del Monte)	2 fl oz	20	0	0
*Roja, Mild (Del Monte)	2 fl oz	20	0	0
Sloppy Joe:				
*Mexican (Hunt's)	5 T	40	0	0
*Original (Hunt's)	5 T	40	0	0
Sour Cream (French's)	2-1/2 T	60	5	75
Soy:				
*Shoyu (Store Brand)	2 fl oz	30	0	0
*(Store Brand)	2 fl oz	24	0	0
*(Tamari)	2 fl oz	35	0	0
Spaghetti:				
(Francesco Rinaldi)	4 fl oz	80	4	45
(French's)	5 fl oz	100	4	36
*(Hunt's)	4 fl oz	80	2	22
*(Prego)	4 fl oz	80	2	22
*(Ragu)	4 fl oz	70	2	26

FOOD	MEASURE OR QUANTITY	CALORIES	FAT GRAMS	% FAT
*(Spatini)	4 fl oz	80	0	0
Thick (French's)	1 cup	170	7	37
Thick and Zesty (Ragu)	4 fl oz	100	4	36
Spaghetti with Meat:				
(Prego)	4 fl oz	150	6	36
(Ragu)	4 fl oz	100	4	36
Spaghetti with Mushrooms:				
(French's)	5 fl oz	100	4	36
(Prego)	4 fl oz	140	5	32
(Ragu)	4 fl oz	110	5	41
Stir-Fry (Kikkoman)	1 T	18	1	50
Stroganoff, Mix (French's)	1/3 cup	110	5	41
Sweet and Sour:				
*(Contadina)	4 fl oz	150	3	18
*(French's)	4 fl oz	55	0	0
(La Choy)	1 T	20	1	45
Taco, Hot:				
*(Del Monte)	2 fl oz	15	0	0
*(Old El Paso)	2 T	11	0	0
Taco, Mild:				
*(Del Monte)	2 fl oz	15	0	0
*(Old El Paso)	2 T	11	0	0
Tartar:				
(Hellman's)	1 T	70	7	90
(Kraft)	1 T	70	7	90
Teriyaki:				
*(French's)	2 T	35	0	0
*(Kikkoman)	1 T	15	0	0
*(La Choy)	1 fl oz	30	0	0
Tomato:				
*(Contadina)	4 fl oz	45	0	0
*(Del Monte)	1 cup	70	1	13
Herb (Hunt's)	4 fl oz	80	4	45
*(Hunt's)	4 fl oz	30	0	0
Special (Hunt's)	4 fl oz	80	4	45
Tomato, Italian Style:				
*(Contadina)	4 fl oz	40	0	0
*(Hunt's)	4 fl oz	60	2	30
***Tomato with Bits** (Hunt's)	4 fl oz	30	0	0
***Tomato with Cheese** (Hunt's)	4 fl oz	45	1	20
***Tomato with Mushrooms** (Hunt's)	4 fl oz	25	0	0
Tomato with Onions:				
*(Del Monte)	4 fl oz	50	0	0
*(Hunt's)	4 fl oz	40	0	0
Welsh Rarebit (Snow's)	4 fl oz	170	11	58
Worcestershire:				
*(Lea & Perrins)	1 T	60	0	0
*(French's)	1 T	10	0	0
*Smoky (French's)	1 T	10	0	0

17. ITALIAN CUISINE

■ ITALIAN CUISINE

SEE ADDITIONAL CHOICES IN GRAVIES AND SAUCES, PASTA DISHES, PIZZA, FROZEN FOODS, AND FAST-FOOD RESTAURANTS
Fat Range = 0% to 90%
Average Fat = 34%

FOOD	MEASURE OR QUANTITY	CALORIES	FAT GRAMS	% FAT
Caesar Salad (Homemade)	2 cups	400	40	90
Cheese Canneloni				
(Lean Cuisine)	1	270	10	33
Cheese Manicotti				
(Budget Gourmet)	1	450	25	50
*Cheese Ravioli Slim Selections				
(Budget Gourmet)	1	260	7	24
Chicken Cacciatore:				
*(Armour Lite)	1	250	4	14
*(Banquet)	1	260	5	17
(Budget Gourmet)	1	300	13	39
(Lean Cuisine)	1	280	10	32
Chicken Marsala:				
*Breast (Armour Lite)	1	250	5	18
*(Classic Lite)	1	270	7	23
*Chicken Milan (Armour)	1	320	10	28
*Chicken Milan (Armour)	1	320	10	28
Chicken Parmigiana:				
Breast (Le Menu)	1	400	20	45
(Homemade)	6 oz	700	30	39
(Hungry-Man)	1	820	52	57
*(Light & Elegant)	1	260	6	21
*Chicken Pasta Divan (Healthy				
Choice)	1	310	4	12
*Chicken and Vermicelli				
(Lean Cuisine)	1	270	7	23
Eggplant Parmigiana				
(Homemade)	6 oz	750	35	42
*Fettucini Slim Selections				
(Budget Gourmet)	1	300	10	30
Fish and Pasta Florentine				
(Mrs. Paul's)	1	240	9	34
Garlic Bread (Homemade)	2 slices	135	12	80
Lasagna:				
(Budget Gourmet)	1	420	20	43
*(Homemade)	6 oz	750	25	30
(Hungry-Man)	1	420	20	43
*(Light & Elegant)	1	280	5	16
*Slim Selections				
(Budget Gourmet)	1	300	10	30

FOOD	MEASURE OR QUANTITY	CALORIES	FAT GRAMS	% FAT
(Swanson)	1	420	19	41
With Meat (Hungry-Man)	1	680	24	32
*Lentil Soup (Homemade)	1 cup	150	3	18
Linguni & Scallops Slim Selections				
(Budget Gourmet)	1	280	11	35
Linguni & Shrimp				
(Budget Gourmet)	1	330	15	41
Macaroni & Beef (Swanson)	1	370	15	36
Macaroni and Cheese:				
(Banquet)	1	230	8	31
(Swanson)	1	380	15	36
Meatball Stew (Lean Cuisine)	1	250	10	36
*Minestrone Soup (Homemade)	1 cup	100	2	18
*Noodles and Chicken (Swanson)	1	270	9	30
*Pasta and Sauce (Banquet)	1	300	8	24
Pasta Shells and Beef				
(Budget Gourmet)	1	340	15	40
Pasta with Vegetables and Ham				
(Lean Cuisine)	1	280	13	42
*Pizza, Cheese (Kid Cuisine)	1	240	4	15
*Ravioli, Mini, Cheese (Kid Cuisine)	1	250	2	7
*Red Snapper ,Dry (Homemade)	6 oz	250	4	14
*Red Snapper with Butter (Homemade)	6 oz	350	10	26
Rigatoni (Lean Cuisine)	1	260	10	35
Scungilli Calamari Salad	4 oz	300	30	90
*Shrimp Cocktail	4	100	0	0
*Shrimp Primavera (Right Choice)	1	240	7	26
*Shrimp Scampi (Homemade)	6 oz	500	15	27
Spaghetti and Meatballs:				
*(Lean Cuisine)	1	280	7	22
(Swanson)	1	410	14	31
*Turkey Parmesan (Classic Lite)	1	240	8	30
Turkey Tetrazzini:				
*(Banquet)	1	270	4	13
*(Morton)	1	280	4	13
*Veal Marsala (Le Menu Light)	1	260	6	21
Veal Parmigiana:				
(Banquet)	1	230	11	43
(Hungry-Man)	1	560	25	40
(Swanson)	1	480	25	47
Veal Scallopini (Homemade)	6 oz	650	40	55

18. JUICES

■ FRUIT JUICES

SEE REFERENCES IN BEVERAGES UNDER FRUIT DRINKS

Fat Range = 0% to 9%

Average Fat = 1%

FOOD	MEASURE OR QUANTITY	CALORIES	FAT GRAMS	% FAT
*Acerola, Fresh Squeezed	6 fl oz	40	0	0
*Apple Grape, Frozen Prepared				
(Welch's)	6 fl oz	90	0	0
*Apple (Mott's)	6 fl oz	80	0	0
*Apricot Nectar	6 fl oz	100	0	0
*Apricot Nectar (Del Monte)	6 fl oz	100	0	0
*Cranberry, Bottle (Ocean Spray)	6 fl oz	110	0	0
*Cranberry, Low Calorie				
(Ocean Spray)	6 fl oz	35	0	0
*Fruit Blend, Frozen Prepared				
(Welch's)	6 fl oz	90	0	0
Grape:				
*(Tang)	6 fl oz	90	0	0
*(Welch's)	6 fl oz	90	0	0
Grape, Frozen Prepared:				
*(Minute Maid)	6 fl oz	100	1	9
*(Welch's)	6 fl oz	100	0	0
*Grape, Sparkling Red (Welch's)	6 fl oz	120	0	0
*Grape, Sparkling White				
(Welch's)	6 fl oz	120	0	0
Grapefruit:				
*(Ocean Spray)	6 fl oz	60	0	0
*(Tang)	6 fl oz	90	0	0
*Grapefruit, Canned Natural				
(Del Monte)	6 fl oz	60	0	0
Grapefruit, Frozen Prepared				
*(Minute Maid)	6 fl oz	75	0	0
*(Ocean Spray)	6 fl oz	70	0	0
*Grapefruit, Fresh Squeezed	6 fl oz	60	0	0
*Lemon (Realemon)	1 T	3	0	0
*Lemon, Fresh Squeezed	6 fl oz	45	0	0
*Lemon Frozen Prepared				
(Minute Maid)	6 fl oz	45	0	0
*Lime (Realime)	1 T	2	0	0
*Lime, Fresh Squeezed	6 fl oz	45	0	0
*Orange, Canned Unsweetened				
(Del Monte)	6 fl oz	80	0	0
Orange, Container:				
*(Minute Maid)	6 fl oz	85	1	11
*With Pulp (Store Brand)	6 fl oz	85	0	0
*Orange, Fresh Squeezed	6 fl oz	80	0	0

FOOD	MEASURE OR QUANTITY	CALORIES	FAT GRAMS	% FAT
*Orange, Frozen Prepared				
(Ocean Spray)	6 fl oz	90	1	10
Orange, Imitation:				
*Awake (Bird's Eye)	6 fl oz	80	0	0
*Plus (Bird's Eye)	6 fl oz	100	0	0
*Orange (Tang)	6 fl oz	90	0	0
*Papaya Nectar	6 fl oz	105	0	0
*Passion, Fresh Squeezed	6 fl oz	115	0	0
*Peach Nectar	6 fl oz	110	0	0
*Pineapple, Canned Unsweetened				
(Del Monte)	6 fl oz	100	0	0
*Prune (Mott's)	6 fl oz	120	0	0
*Prune, Unsweetened				
(Del Monte)	6 fl oz	100	0	0
*Tangerine, Fresh Squeezed	6 fl oz	75	0	0

■ VEGETABLE JUICES
Fat Range = 0%
Average Fat = 0%

FOOD	MEASURE OR QUANTITY	CALORIES	FAT GRAMS	% FAT
*Beefamotto (Mott's)	6 fl oz	80	0	0
*Carrot (Store Brand)	6 fl oz	70	0	0
*Clamatto (Mott's)	6 fl oz	80	0	0
*Tomato (Store Brand)	6 fl oz	30	0	0
*V8 (Campbell's)	6 fl oz	40	0	0
*Vegetable	6 fl oz	35	0	0

19. WEIGHT-LOSS AIDS

■ BREAKFAST AND DIET BARS
Fat Range = 26% to 52%
Average Fat = 45%

FOOD	MEASURE OR QUANTITY	CALORIES	FAT GRAMS	% FAT
Chocolate:				
Diet Bar (Carnation)	2	270	14	47

FOOD	MEASURE OR QUANTITY	CALORIES	FAT GRAMS	% FAT
Figurine (Pillsbury)	1	100	5	45
*(Slim Fast)	1	130	4	28
Chocolate Caramel, Figurine (Pillsbury)	1	100	5	45
Chocolate Chip, Breakfast (Carnation)	1	200	11	50
Chocolate Crunch, Breakfast (Carnation)	1	190	10	47
Chocolate Peanut Butter:				
Diet Bar (Carnation)	2	270	15	50
Figurine (Pillsbury)	1	100	5	45
Honey Nut, Breakfast (Carnation)	1	190	11	52
*Peanut Butter (Slim Fast)	1	140	4	26
Peanut Butter, Crunch (Carnation)	1	200	11	50
Peanut Butter with Chocolate Chips (Carnation)	1	200	11	50
S'More, Figurine (Pillsbury)	1	100	5	45
Vanilla:				
Diet Bar (Carnation)	2	270	15	50
Figurine (Pillsbury)	1	100	5	45

■ MEDICALLY SUPERVISED SUPPLEMENTS

Fat Range = 0% to 18%
Average Fat = 0%

FOOD	MEASURE OR QUANTITY	CALORIES	FAT GRAMS	% FAT
*Complement 100	1	104	0	0
*Complement 100	5	520	1	2
*HMR 500	1	104	0	0
*HMR 500	5	520	1	2
*HMR 70	1	104	0	0
*HMR 70	5	520	3	5
*HMR Chicken	5	510	5	9
*HMR Chicken	1	102	1	9
*Medifast	1	87	0	0
*Medifast	5	435	1	2
*Nutrimed 420	1	84	0	0
*Nutrimed 420	5	420	1	2
*Optifast 45	1	60	0	0
*Optifast 45	5	300	0	0
*Optifast 70	1	65	0	0
*Optifast 70	5	420	2	4
*Pro Cal	1	103	2	18
*Pro Cal	5	515	10	17

■ OVER-THE-COUNTER FOOD SUPPLEMENTS
Fat Range = 5% to 16%
Average Fat = 13%

FOOD	MEASURE OR QUANTITY	CALORIES	FAT GRAMS	% FAT
*Banana, Slender (Carnation)	10 fl oz	220	4	16
Chocolate:				
*Slender (Carnation)	10 fl oz	220	4	16
*(Slim Fast)[1]	1 oz	190	1	5
*Ultra (Slim Fast)[1]	1 oz	220	3	12
*Chocolate Fudge, Slender (Carnation)	10 fl oz	220	4	16
*Chocolate Malted, Slender (Carnation)	10 fl oz	220	4	16
*Chocolate, Milk, Slender (Carnation)	10 fl oz	220	4	16
*Peach, Slender (Carnation)	10 fl oz	220	4	16
Strawberry:				
*(Slim Fast)[1]	1 oz	190	1	5
*Ultra (Slim Fast)[1]	1 oz	220	3	12
Vanilla:				
*Slender (Carnation)	10 fl oz	220	4	16
*(Slim Fast)[1]	1 oz	190	1	5
*Ultra (Slim Fast)[1]	1 oz	220	3	12

20. MEATS

■ BEEF CUTS
Fat Range = 26% to 84%
Average Fat = 56%

FOOD	MEASURE OR QUANTITY	CALORIES	FAT GRAMS	% FAT
Brisket:				
Point Half, Lean and Fat	3 oz	310	25	73
Whole, Lean and Fat	3 oz	330	30	82
Chuck Arm Pot Roast, Lean and Fat	3 oz	300	22	66
Chuck Blade Roast:				
Choice Grade, Lean and Fat	3 oz	330	25	68

[1]Prepared with 8 ounces of skim milk.

FOOD	MEASURE OR QUANTITY	CALORIES	FAT GRAMS	% FAT
Lean and Fat	3 oz	325	25	69
Prime Grade,				
Lean and Fat	3 oz	350	30	77
Corned Beef Brisket	3 oz	215	16	67
Corned Beef Brisket, Cured	3 oz	220	18	74
Flank, Choice Grade, Lean and				
Fat	3 oz	215	12	50
Ground Beef, Lean:				
17% Fat	3 oz	210	14	60
17% Fat, Pan Fried	3 oz	225	14	56
21% Fat, Baked	3 oz	230	16	63
21% Fat, Pan Fried	3 oz	234	16	62
27% Fat, Baked	3 oz	240	18	68
27% Fat, Pan Fried	3 oz	260	19	66
Rib:				
Large End, Rib 6–9, Broiled	3 oz	320	30	84
Small End, Rib 10–12, Broiled	3 oz	280	21	68
Whole, Rib 6–12, Broiled	3 oz	300	25	75
Round Bottom:				
Lean, Braised	3 oz	190	8	38
Lean and Fat, Braised	3 oz	220	13	53
Round Eye:				
Lean, Roasted	3 oz	155	7	41
Lean and Fat, Roasted	3 oz	200	12	54
Round Full Cut:				
Lean, Roasted	3 oz	165	7	38
Lean and Fat, Roasted	3 oz	230	16	63
Round Tip:				
Lean, Roasted	3 oz	160	6	34
Lean and Fat, Roasted	3 oz	214	13	55
Round Top:				
*Lean, Broiled	3 oz	160	5	28
Lean and Fat, Broiled	3 oz	180	7	35
Shank Crosscuts:				
*Lean, Simmered	3 oz	170	5	26
Lean and Fat, Simmered	3 oz	210	10	43
Shortloin Porterhouse:				
Lean, Broiled	3 oz	185	9	44
Lean and Fat, Broiled	3 oz	260	18	62
Shortribs:				
Lean, Braised	3 oz	250	15	54
Lean and Fat, Braised	3 oz	220	13	53
T-Bone Steak:				
Lean, Broiled	3 oz	180	9	45
Lean and Fat, Broiled	3 oz	280	21	68
Tenderloin:				
Lean, Broiled	3 oz	175	8	41
Lean and Fat, Broiled	3 oz	230	15	59
Top Loin:				
Lean, Broiled	3 oz	170	8	42
Lean and Fat, Broiled	3 oz	240	16	60
Wedge Bone Sirloin:				
Lean, Broiled	3 oz	180	7	35
Lean and Fat, Broiled	3 oz	240	15	56

■ BEEF GRAVY
Fat Range = 36%
Average Fat = 36%

FOOD	MEASURE OR QUANTITY	CALORIES	FAT GRAMS	% FAT
(Franco-American)	2 oz	25	1	36

■ BEEF ORGANS
Fat Range = 22% to 70%
Average Fat = 46%

FOOD	MEASURE OR QUANTITY	CALORIES	FAT GRAMS	% FAT
Brain, Pan Fried	3 oz	170	13	69
***Heart,** Simmered	3 oz	150	5	30
***Kidneys,** Simmered	3 oz	120	3	22
***Liver,** Braised	3 oz	140	4	26
***Lungs,** Simmered	3 oz	100	3	27
Pancreas, Braised	3 oz	230	15	59
Thymus, Cooked	3 oz	270	21	70
Tongue, Simmered	3 oz	250	18	65
Tripe, Cooked	3 oz	100	5	45

■ CALF ORGANS
Fat Range = 16% to 65%
Average Fat = 43%

FOOD	MEASURE OR QUANTITY	CALORIES	FAT GRAMS	% FAT
Brain, Braised	3-½ oz	125	9	65
Liver, Fried	3-½ oz	260	14	48
***Sweetbread,** Braised	3-½ oz	170	3	16

■ LAMB CUTS
Fat Range = 34% to 77%
Average Fat = 55%

FOOD	MEASURE OR QUANTITY	CALORIES	FAT GRAMS	% FAT
Leg:				
Lean, Roasted	3 oz	160	6	34
Lean and Fat, Roasted	3 oz	237	16	61

FOOD	MEASURE OR QUANTITY	CALORIES	FAT GRAMS	% FAT
Loin Chop:				
Lean, Roasted	3 oz	160	6	34
Lean and Fat, Roasted	3 oz	305	25	74
Rib Chop:				
Lean, Broiled	3 oz	180	9	45
Lean and Fat, Broiled	3 oz	350	30	77
Shoulder:				
Lean, Roasted	3 oz	175	9	46
Lean and Fat, Roasted	3 oz	290	23	71

■ LUNCHEON MEATS
Fat Range = 26% to 90%
Average Fat = 70%

FOOD	MEASURE OR QUANTITY	CALORIES	FAT GRAMS	% FAT
Bacon (Oscar Meyer)	1	39	3	69
Bacon, Canadian:				
*(Light & Lean)	2	35	1	26
*(Oscar Meyer)	1	35	1	26
Beef, Breakfast Strip				
(Lean & Tasty)	1	46	4	78
Beef, Chopped				
(Armour)	3 oz	280	24	77
Beef Smokies				
(Oscar Meyer)	1	122	11	81
Bockwurst				
(Store Brand)	1	200	19	86
Bologna:				
(Ball Park)	1 slice	110	10	82
(Hormel)	2	170	16	85
Bologna, Beef:				
(Armour)	1 oz	90	8	80
(Oscar Meyer)	1	74	7	85
(Store Brand)	1	70	7	90
Bologna, Beef and Pork				
(Store Brand)	1	70	7	90
Bologna, Cheese				
(Oscar Meyer)	1	75	7	84
Bologna, Pork				
(Store Brand)	1	70	7	90
Bologna, Thin Sliced				
(Light & Lean)	2	70	6	77
Bratwurst (Store Brand)	1 oz	90	8	80
Braunschweiger (Hormel)	1 oz	80	7	79
Brotwurst (Store Brand)	1	230	20	78
Capocollo (Hormel)	1 oz	80	6	68
Corned Beef:				
(Dinty Moore)	2 oz	130	8	55
(Oscar Meyer)	1 sl	24	1	38
(Store Brand)	1 oz	60	3	45

FOOD	MEASURE OR QUANTITY	CALORIES	FAT GRAMS	% FAT
Frankfurter:				
(Armour)	1	170	15	79
(Ball Park)	1	175	17	87
Deli (Hebrew National)	2.3 oz	200	19	86
(Hebrew National)	1.6 oz	140	13	84
(Hebrew National)	1.8 oz	160	15	84
(Oscar Meyer)	1.6 oz	144	13	81
(Oscar Meyer)	2 oz	190	17	81
(Oscar Meyer)	2.7 oz	230	21	82
Frankfurter, Bacon and Cheese				
(Oscar Meyer)	1	143	14	88
Frankfurter, Beef:				
Jumbo (Armour)	1	190	18	85
(Store Brand)	1	180	16	80
Ham, Barbecue (Light & Lean)	2	50	2	36
Ham and Cheese Loaf				
(Light & Lean)	2	90	6	60
(Oscar Meyer)	1 oz	76	6	71
Ham, Chunk (Hormel)	7 oz	320	21	59
Ham, Cooked (Light & Lean)	2	50	2	36
Ham, Cured:				
Lean (Store Brand)	1	35	2	51
Regular (Store Brand)	1	55	3	49
Ham, Deviled (Armour)	3 oz	140	14	90
***Ham, Honey** (Oscar Meyer)	1	30	1	30
Ham, Italian Style				
(Oscar Meyer)	1	22	1	41
***Ham, Low Salt** (Armour)	1 oz	35	1	26
Ham, Prosciutto (Hormel)	1 oz	90	7	70
Ham, Smoked (Oscar Meyer)	1	23	1	39
Headcheese:				
(Oscar Meyer)	1	55	4	65
(Store Brand)	1	60	5	75
Hot Dog (See Frankfurter)				
Kielbasa:				
Skinless (Hormel)	1	360	26	65
(Store Brand)	1 oz	90	8	80
Knockwurst (Ball Park)	1	335	31	83
Kolbase, Sausage (Hormel)	3 oz	220	19	78
Liver, Pâté (Store Brand)	1 oz	100	8	72
Liverwurst:				
(Hormel)	1 oz	80	7	79
Spread (Hormel)	1 T	40	3	68
Olive Loaf:				
(Hormel)	2	100	7	63
(Store Brand)	1	70	5	64
Pastrami, Beef				
(Store Brand)	1 oz	100	8	72
Pepperoni (Hormel)	1 oz	140	13	84
Pork, Breakfast Strip				
(Lean & Tasty)	1	52	5	87
Salami, Beef:				
Beer (Oscar Meyer)	1	70	6	77
and Pork (Store Brand)	1	80	7	79
Salami Cotto				
(Oscar Meyer)	1	45	3	60

FOOD	MEASURE OR QUANTITY	CALORIES	FAT GRAMS	% FAT
Salami, Genoa:				
(Hormel)	1 oz	110	10	82
(Oscar Meyer)	1	35	3	77
Salami, Hard (Hormel)	2	80	7	79
Salami, Low Salt (Armour)	1 oz	80	7	79
Salami, Piccolo (Hormel)	1 oz	120	11	82
Sausage, Breakfast Patties				
(Jones)	1	135	11	73
Sausage, Brown 'n Serve				
(Hormel)	2	140	13	84
Sausage, Grillers				
(Morningstar Farms)	1	190	13	62
Sausage, Italian Style				
(Store Brand)	1	220	18	74
Sausage Links:				
Brown 'n Serve (Jones)	1	136	11	73
(Morningstar Farms)	3	200	14	63
Pork, Light Breakfast (Jones)	1	55	5	82
Sausage, Little Friers				
(Oscar Meyer)	1	77	7	82
Sausage, Little Smokies				
(Oscar Meyer)	1	30	3	90
Sausage, New England Style				
(Oscar Meyer)	1	30	2	60
Sausage Patties				
(Morningstar Farms)	2	220	14	57
Sausage, Polish (Store Brand)	1 oz	90	8	80
Sausage, Smoked:				
(Oscar Meyer)	1	124	11	80
(Store Brand)	1	270	21	70
Sausage, Vienna (Armour)	1	200	18	81
Spam:				
Deviled (Hormel)	1 T	40	3	68
Cheese (Hormel)	2 oz	170	16	85
Thuringer, Beef and Pork				
(Store Brand)	1	70	6	77 .
Wiener (See Frankfurter)				

■ **PORK CUTS**
Fat Range = 26% to 94%
Average Fat = 59%

FOOD	MEASURE OR QUANTITY	CALORIES	FAT GRAMS	% FAT
Arm Picnic:				
Lean, Braised	3 oz	210	10	43
Lean and Fat, Braised	3 oz	295	22	67
Lean and Fat, Cured	3 oz	238	18	68
Bacon	3 slices	100	9	81
Blade Roll, Lean & Fat, Cured	3 oz	240	20	75

FOOD	MEASURE OR QUANTITY	CALORIES	FAT GRAMS	% FAT
Boston Blade:				
Lean, Braised	3 oz	250	15	54
Lean and Fat, Braised	3 oz	320	24	68
Chitterlings, Cooked	3 oz	260	24	83
Ears, Cooked	1 ear	180	12	60
Fat, Cooked	1 oz	200	21	94
Ham, Boneless:				
Lean, Roasted	3 oz	140	7	45
Regular 11% Fat, Roasted	3 oz	150	8	48
Ham Leg Rump Half:				
Lean, Roasted	3 oz	190	9	43
Lean and Fat, Roasted	3 oz	230	15	59
Ham Leg Shank Half				
Lean, Roasted	3 oz	180	9	45
Lean and Fat, Roasted	3 oz	260	20	69
Ham Leg Whole				
Lean, Roasted	3 oz	190	9	43
Lean and Fat, Roasted	3 oz	250	18	65
Ham Whole:				
Lean, Roasted	3 oz	130	5	35
Lean and Fat, Roasted	3 oz	200	14	63
Ham, Canned, Roasted	3 oz	140	7	45
Loin Blade:				
Lean, Braised	3 oz	265	18	61
Lean and Fat, Braised	3 oz	350	29	75
Loin Center:				
Lean, Braised	3 oz	230	12	47
Lean and Fat, Braised	3 oz	300	22	66
Rib Center:				
Lean, Braised	3 oz	230	12	47
Lean and Fat, Braised	3 oz	312	23	66
Sirloin:				
Lean, Braised	3 oz	220	11	45
Lean and Fat, Braised	3 oz	230	22	86
Spareribs, Lean and Fat	3 oz	340	25	66
***Tenderloin,** Lean and Fat, Roasted	3 oz	140	4	26
Top Loin:				
Lean, Braised	3 oz	240	12	45
Lean and Fat, Braised	3 oz	320	25	70
Whole:				
Lean, Braised	3 oz	230	12	47
Lean and Fat, Braised	3 oz	310	24	70

■ **PORK ORGANS**
Fat Range = 21% to 79%
Average Fat = 54%

FOOD	MEASURE OR QUANTITY	CALORIES	FAT GRAMS	% FAT
*Spleen, Braised	3 oz	130	3	21
Tail, Braised	3 oz	340	30	79
Tongue, Braised	3 oz	230	16	63

■ **VEAL CUTS**
Fat Range = 25% to 62%
Average Fat = 47%

FOOD	MEASURE OR QUANTITY	CALORIES	FAT GRAMS	% FAT
Breast, Stewed	3 oz	260	18	62
Chuck Cuts, Boneless, Stewed	3 oz	200	11	50
Loin, Broiled	3 oz	200	11	50
Rib Roast, Baked	3 oz	230	14	55
Roasts, Leg and Cutlets, Broiled	3 oz	185	9	44
*Steak, Cooked	3 oz	110	3	25

21. MEXICAN CUISINE

■ **MEXICAN CUISINE**
MORE CHOICES IN GRAVIES AND SAUCES, FROZEN FOODS, AND FAST-FOOD RESTAURANTS
Fat Range = 9% to 82%
Average Fat = 40%

FOOD	MEASURE OR QUANTITY	CALORIES	FAT GRAMS	% FAT
Burrito:				
*Beef and Bean (Patio)	5 oz	320	9	25
Beef and Cheese (Swanson)	1	700	30	39
Beef, Red Hot (El Charrito)	5 oz	340	17	45
Beefsteak (Weight Watchers)	1	330	12	33
Chicken (Weight Watchers)	1	330	14	38

FOOD	MEASURE OR QUANTITY	CALORIES	FAT GRAMS	% FAT
Chili and Beef (Patio)	5 oz	330	13	35
Crispy Fried				
(Van de Kamp's)	6 oz	430	16	33
Burrito Dinner:				
*(Patio)	1	517	16	28
(Swanson)	1	720	32	40
Green Chili (El Charrito)	5 oz	370	16	39
Jalapeño (El Charrito)	6 oz	410	15	33
Red Hot:				
(El Charrito)	5 oz	375	18	43
(Patio)	5 oz	350	15	39
Chili, Beef and Bean				
(Patio)	5 oz	330	12	33
Chili Con Carne:				
Canned (Heinz)	8 oz	350	21	54
(Van de Kamp's)	8 oz	410	36	79
Chili Con Carne, with Beans:				
Frozen (Stouffer's)	8 oz	280	11	35
Hot (Heinz)	8 oz	330	16	44
(Van de Kamp's)	8 oz	350	23	59
(Wolf's)	8 oz	345	22	57
Chimichanca:				
Beef (El Paso)	1	380	23	54
Chicken (El Paso)	1	370	21	51
Enchilada:				
Beef:				
*(Banquet)	1	500	15	27
(Patio)	1	514	24	42
(Swanson)	1	480	24	45
(Van de Kamp's)	1	390	15	35
Beef and Cheese				
(Van de Kamp's)	1	540	20	33
Beef Suiza				
(Weight Watchers)	1	310	13	38
Cheese:				
(Banquet)	1	540	19	32
(El Charrito)	1	570	24	38
*(Patio)	1	380	9	21
Ranchero (Weight Watchers)	1	370	22	54
*Chicken (El Charrito)	1	510	17	30
Fajitas:				
*Beef (Weight Watchers)	1	270	7	23
*Chicken (Weight Watchers)	1	260	6	21
Guacamole (Kraft)	1 oz	110	10	82
Mexican Dinner:				
(Banquet)	1	480	18	34
*Combination (Banquet)	1	520	17	29
(El Charrito)	1	700	35	45
(Patio)	1	530	24	41
*Queso (El Charrito)	1	490	16	29
Ranchero Dinner (Patio)	1	470	21	40
Taco:				
Beef (Patio)	2	240	9	34
Beef and Chili Beans (Patio)	11 oz	640	32	45
Plain (El Paso)	1	50	2	36

FOOD	MEASURE OR QUANTITY	CALORIES	FAT GRAMS	% FAT
Taco Shell (Ortega)	1	50	2	36
Tortilla:				
*Flour (El Charrito)	2	170	4	21
*Frozen (Patio)	2	100	1	9
Tostada, Beef (Van de Kamp's)	8-½ oz	530	30	51

22. NUTS AND SEEDS

■ **NUTS**
Fat Range = 0% to 90%
Average Fat = 68%

FOOD	MEASURE OR QUANTITY	CALORIES	FAT GRAMS	% FAT
Almond, Butter	1 T	118	10	76
Almonds:				
Chopped	1 cup	824	68	74
Slivers	1 cup	728	60	74
Almonds, Barbecue				
(Blue Diamond)	1 oz	150	15	90
Almonds, Cheese				
(Blue Diamond)	1 oz	140	12	77
Almonds, Hickory Smoke Dry				
Roasted (Blue Diamond)	1 oz	150	13	78
Almonds, Smokehouse (Blue				
Diamond)	1 oz	150	14	84
Beechnuts	1 oz	192	16	75
Brazil Nuts	1 cup	989	93	85
Butter Nuts	1 oz	184	16	78
Cashews, Dried	1 cup	840	64	69
Cashews, Honey Roasted				
(Planters)	1 oz	170	12	64
Cashews, Oil Roasted	1 cup	799	63	71
Cashews and Peanuts, Honey				
Roasted (Planters)	1 oz	170	12	64
Chestnuts:				
*Chinese, Boiled	1 oz	70	0	0
*Chinese, Dried	1 oz	100	1	9
*European, Boiled	1 oz	50	1	18
*Japanese, Boiled	1 oz	16	0	0
*Japanese, Dried	1 oz	100	0	0

FOOD	MEASURE OR QUANTITY	CALORIES	FAT GRAMS	% FAT
Coconut Cream:				
Plain (Raw)	1 cup	847	83	88
Sweetened (Coco Loco)	1 cup	600	53	80
Coconut, Dried	1 cup	485	33	61
Coconut Flakes	1 cup	356	24	61
Coconut Milk (Raw)	1 cup	589	57	87
Coconut Milk	1 T	100	9	81
Coconut Milk, Condensed	1 cup	445	48	97
Coconut Shredded (Baker's)	3 oz	140	10	64
Coconut Shredded	1 cup	303	27	80
Filbert Nuts	1 cup	780	72	83
Filberts Roasted (Blue Diamond)	1 oz	166	15	81
*****Ginko**	1 oz	32	1	28
Hickory	1 oz	198	18	82
Macadamia:				
Dry Roasted	1 cup	998	98	88
Oil Roasted	1 cup	1031	103	90
Mixed Nuts, Dry Roasted	1 cup	875	71	73
Mixed Nuts, Dry Roasted				
(Planters)	1 oz	170	15	79
Mixed Nuts, Oil Roasted	1 cup	936	80	77
Mixed Nuts, Oil Roasted,				
Deluxe (Planters)	1 oz	180	17	85
Mixed Nuts, Oil Roasted				
(Planters)	1 oz	180	16	80
Nut Topping (Planters)	1 oz	170	15	79
Peanut Butter, Chunky:				
(Jiffy)	1 T	75	8	96
(Skippy)	1 T	75	8	96
(Store Brand)	1 T	100	8	72
(Store Brand)	1 cup	1629	129	71
Peanut Butter, Creamy:				
(Jiffy)	1 T	75	8	96
(Skippy)	1 T	75	8	96
(Store Brand)	1 T	104	8	69
Peanuts, Dry Roasted Lite				
(Planters)	1 oz	164	14	77
Peanuts, Oil Roasted	1 cup	903	71	71
Peanuts, Roasted in Shell				
(Store Brand)	10	110	9	74
Pecan Halves, Dry Roasted	1 cup	769	73	85
Pecans, Oil Roasted	1 cup	806	78	87
Persia Nuts	1 cup	822	74	81
Pignoli Nuts, Dried	1 oz	150	14	84
Pine Nuts, Dried	1 oz	150	14	84
Pistachio Nuts, Dry Roasted				
(Blue Diamond)	50	130	12	83
Pistachio Nuts, Red Roasted	1 cup	828	68	74
Redskin, Oil Roasted (Planters)	1 oz	170	15	79
Soybeans, Oil Roasted	1 cup	526	26	44
Spanish, Dry Roasted	1 cup	892	72	73
Tavern Nuts (Planters)	1 oz	170	15	79
Walnuts, Black	1 cup	525	45	77
Walnuts Halves	1 cup	650	65	90
Walnuts, Chopped	1 cup	800	80	90

FOOD	MEASURE OR QUANTITY	CALORIES	FAT GRAMS	% FAT
Trail Mix:				
Deluxe Mixture (Carnation)	1 pkg	130	8	55
*Nut & Fruit Mixture (Carnation)	1 pkg	100	3	27
Nut 'n Fruit Mix (Planters)	1 oz	150	9	54
Raisin and Nut Mixture (Carnation)	1 pkg	130	7	48

■ **SEEDS**
Fat Range = 14% to 87% Fat
Average Fat = 70%

FOOD	MEASURE OR QUANTITY	CALORIES	FAT GRAMS	% FAT
*Breadfruit	1 cup	65	1	14
Lotus Seeds, Dried	1 oz	95	8	76
Pumpkin:				
Dried	1 oz	155	13	75
Hulled	1 cup	803	63	71
Roasted	1 oz	150	12	72
Safflower, Dried	1 oz	150	11	66
Sesame	1 cup	884	72	73
Sesame Butter Tahini	1 T	90	8	80
Sesame Dried	1 oz	50	4	72
Sesame Nut Mix:				
Dry Roasted (Planters)	1 oz	160	12	68
Oil Roasted (Planters)	1 oz	160	13	73
Sesame, Toasted	1 oz	170	14	74
Squash, Dried	1 oz	155	13	75
Sunflower, Hulled	1 cup	879	71	73
Sunflower, Hulled, Dried	1 oz	170	14	74
Sunflower, Oil Roasted	1 oz	175	17	87
Watermelon, Dried	1 oz	158	13	74

23. ORIENTAL CUISINE

■ ORIENTAL CUISINE
MORE CHOICES IN RICE, RICE DISHES, AND FROZEN FOODS
Fat Range = 6% to 62%
Average Fat = 22%

FOOD	MEASURE OR QUANTITY	CALORIES	FAT GRAMS	% FAT
*Beef Broccoli (La Choy)	11 oz	290	7	22
Beef Chop Suey (Stouffer's)	1	340	12	32
Beef Chow Mein:				
(Chung King)	1	290	20	62
*(Van de Kamp's)	1	310	10	29
Beef, Oriental:				
*(Lean Cuisine)	1	270	8	27
*Slim Selections				
(Budget Gourmet)	1	300	9	27
Beef Pepper Oriental:				
*(Healthy Choice)	1	290	6	19
*(La Choy)	6 fl oz	80	1	11
Beef Teriyaki:				
*(La Choy)	10 oz	280	7	22
*(Light & Elegant)	1	240	3	11
Chicken Chow Mein:				
*(Chun King)	1	230	5	20
*(Classic Lite)	1	220	4	16
*(La Choy)	1	260	4	14
*(La Choy)	6 fl oz	90	2	20
(Stouffer's)	1	140	5	32
*Chicken Hawaiian (Armour)	1	280	5	16
*Chicken Imperial				
(Weight Watchers)	1	230	4	16
Chicken, Mandarin:				
*(Budget Gourmet)	1	290	7	22
*Slim Selections (Budget				
Gourmet)	1	300	6	18
*Chicken, Orange (Lean Cuisine)	1	270	5	17
Chicken, Oriental:				
*(Armour Lite)	1	250	4	14
*(Classic Lite)	1	250	6	22
*(Healthy Choice)	1	220	2	8
Chicken, Sweet and Sour:				
*(Armour Lite)	1	240	2	8
*(Budget Gourmet)	1	350	7	18
*(Classic Lite)	1	250	3	11
*(Healthy Choice)	1	280	2	6
*(La Choy)	10 oz	280	4	13
(Le Menu)	1	450	22	44
(Weight Watchers)	1	460	22	43

FOOD	MEASURE OR QUANTITY	CALORIES	FAT GRAMS	% FAT
Chicken Teriyaki				
(Dinner Classic)	1	340	15	40
Egg Roll:				
Beef (La Choy)	2	380	13	31
Chicken Almond (La Choy)	2	450	20	40
*Lobster (La Choy)	1	180	5	25
*Shrimp (La Choy)	1	160	4	22
***Shrimp Chow Mein** (La Choy)	6 fl oz	70	1	13
***Shrimp with Lobster Sauce**				
(La Choy)	10 oz	220	7	29

24. PIZZA

■ PIZZA
ALSO SEE FAST-FOOD RESTAURANTS
Fat Range = 12% to 57%
Average Fat = 42%

FOOD	MEASURE OR QUANTITY	CALORIES	FAT GRAMS	% FAT
Cheese:				
(Celeste)	6.5 oz	500	25	45
Extra (Totino)	¼ pie	250	12	43
French Bread (Stouffer's)	5 oz	340	13	34
Heat 'n Eat (Totino)	4 oz	270	11	37
*(Kid's Cuisine)	1	240	4	15
Microwave (Pillsbury)	7 oz	480	19	36
Microwave (Totino)	4 oz	250	9	32
Party (Totino)	⅓ pie	255	12	42
Pizzeria Type	1 slice	500	25	45
Single Serve (Totino)	7 oz	490	21	39
(Totino)	¼ pie	350	15	39
20 ounce (Celeste)	¼ pie	320	16	45
*(Weight Watchers)	6 oz	320	8	22
Combination:				
(Pillsbury)	9 oz	670	36	48
Single Serve (Totino)	9 oz	690	39	51
Deluxe:				
French Bread (Stouffer's)	6 oz	430	21	44
22 Ounce (Celeste)	¼ pie	380	22	52
*(Weight Watchers)	7 oz	300	8	24
French Bread (Weight Watchers)	6 oz	330	12	33

FOOD	MEASURE OR QUANTITY	CALORIES	FAT GRAMS	% FAT
Hamburger, French Bread (Stouffer's)	6 oz	410	18	40
Nacho Pizza (Totino)	1/3 pie	230	13	51
Pepperoni:				
French Bread (Stouffer's)	6 oz	390	18	42
Heat 'n Eat (Totino)	5 oz	350	18	46
(Pillsbury)	9 oz	600	28	42
Single Serve (Totino)	9 oz	610	31	46
10 Ounce (Celeste)	1/4 pie	370	21	51
Pizza Mix:				
*Thick Crust (Contadina)	1/4 pie	300	4	12
*Thin Crust (Contadina)	1/4 pie	200	3	14
Pizza Sauce:				
(Ragu)	3 tbsp	45	2	40
(Store Brand)	4 oz	40	2	45
Sausage:				
French Bread (Stouffer's)	6 oz	420	20	43
Heat 'n Eat (Totino)	5 oz	360	20	50
(Pillsbury)	9 oz	650	34	47
(Pizzeria Type)	6 oz	600	30	45
Single Serve (Totino)	9 oz	660	37	50
(Totino)	1/4 pie	280	16	51
20 Ounce (Celeste)	1/4 pie	380	22	52
Sausage and Mushroom:				
French Bread (Stouffer's)	6 oz	400	17	38
(Pizzeria Type)	6 oz	625	30	43
22 Ounce (Celeste)	1/4 pie	400	22	50
Sausage and Pepperoni				
(Pizzeria Type)	6 oz	625	30	43
Supreme 23 Ounce (Celeste)	1/4 pie	380	24	57

25. POULTRY

■ **CAPON PARTS**
Fat Range = 47% to 57%
Average Fat = 50%

FOOD	MEASURE OR QUANTITY	CALORIES	FAT GRAMS	% FAT
Dark Meat with Skin, Roasted	3-1/2 oz	230	12	47
Light and Dark Meat with Skin,				
Roasted	3-1/2 oz	220	14	57

■ CHICKEN PARTS

Fat Range = 19% to 79%
Average Fat = 46%

FOOD	MEASURE OR QUANTITY	CALORIES	FAT GRAMS	% FAT
Back Half with Skin (Fried)	2-½ oz	240	15	56
Breast Half with Skin:				
Batter Dipped, Fried	3-½ oz	240	11	41
Fried	3-½ oz	220	9	37
Roasted	3-½ oz	190	8	38
Stewed	3-½ oz	200	8	36
Breast Half without Skin:				
*Fried	3-½ oz	160	4	22
*Roasted	3-½ oz	140	3	19
*Stewed	3-½ oz	145	3	19
Chicken with Skin:				
4-½ lb Bird, Roasted	½ bird	1070	65	55
3 lb Bird, Stewed	½ bird	740	50	61
Chicken without Skin:				
4-½ lb Bird, Roasted	½ bird	650	26	36
3 lb Bird, Stewed	½ bird	470	24	46
Dark Meat with Skin:				
Fried	3-½ oz	290	17	53
Fried	1 oz	84	5	54
Roasted	1 oz	71	4	51
Roasted	3-½ oz	250	16	58
Dark Meat Without Skin:				
Fried	1 oz	68	3	40
Fried	3-½ oz	240	12	45
Roasted	3-½ oz	200	10	45
Roasted	1 oz	60	3	45
Stewed	3-½ oz	190	9	43
Drumstick with Skin:				
Batter Dipped, Fried	1	180	9	45
Fried	1	120	7	52
Roasted	1	115	6	47
Stewed	1	115	6	47
Drumstick without Skin:				
Fried	1	100	5	45
*Roasted	1	90	3	30
Stewed	1	80	3	34
Giblets:				
Fried	3-½ oz	280	14	45
*Roasted	3-½ oz	160	5	28
Leg with Skin:				
Batter Dipped, Fried	1	300	18	54
Fried	1	290	17	53
Roasted	1	270	15	50
Stewed	1	275	16	52
Leg Without Skin Stewed	1	190	8	38
Light and Dark Meat with Skin:				
Batter Dipped, Fried	3-½ oz	300	18	54
Flour Coated, Fried	3-½ oz	270	15	50
Light Meat with Skin:				
Fried	3-½ oz	250	12	43

FOOD	MEASURE OR QUANTITY	CALORIES	FAT GRAMS	% FAT
Fried	1 oz	70	4	51
Roasted	3-½ oz	220	11	45
Roasted	1 oz	60	3	45
Stewed	3-½ oz	200	10	45
Light Meat Without Skin:				
*Fried	3-½ oz	190	6	28
Fried	1 oz	55	2	33
Roasted	1 oz	50	2	36
*Roasted	3-½ oz	170	5	26
*Stewed	3-½ oz	160	4	22
Liver, Roasted	3-½ oz	160	6	34
Skin:				
Flour Dipped, Fried	1 oz	170	15	79
Roasted	1 oz	150	12	72
Stewed	1 oz	150	12	72
Thigh with Skin:				
Batter Dipped, Fried	1	190	10	47
Fried	1	160	9	51
Roasted	1	150	10	60
Thigh Without Skin:				
(Roasted)	1	100	6	54
(Stewed)	1	100	6	54
Wing with Skin:				
(Fried)	1	100	6	54
(Roasted)	1	100	6	54

■ CHICKEN, PROCESSED

Fat Range = 0% to 80%
Average Fat = 51%

FOOD	MEASURE OR QUANTITY	CALORIES	FAT GRAMS	% FAT
Breast, Batter Dipped (Weaver)	3-½ oz	250	16	58
Breast, Chunk, Canned:				
(Hormel)	7 oz	350	20	51
(Swanson)	2-½ oz	130	8	55
Breast, Crispy Dutch (Weaver)	3-½ oz	285	18	57
*Breast, Deluxe** (Louis Rich)	1 slice	30	0	0
Breast, Fried (Banquet)	5-¾ oz	218	11	45
*Breast, Hickory Smoked**				
(Weaver)	3-½ oz	125	4	29
*Breast, Oven Roasted** (Weaver)	3-½ oz	120	4	30
Breast Patty:				
And Bun, Microwave, *Hot Bites*				
(Banquet)	4 oz	310	14	41
Hot Bites (Banquet)	2-½ oz	199	12	54
(Tyson)	3 oz	240	17	64
*Breast, Smoked** (Oscar Meyer)	1 slice	26	0	0
Breast, Southern Fried				
Microwave (Banquet)	4 oz	320	14	39

FOOD	MEASURE OR QUANTITY	CALORIES	FAT GRAMS	% FAT
Breast Tenders:				
Hot Bites (Banquet)	2 oz	142	6	38
Hot Bites, Microwave (Banquet)	4 oz	256	10	35
Southern Fried, Microwave (Banquet)	2 oz	155	7	41
Breast (Tyson)	3 oz	190	8	38
Breast with Barbecue Sauce, Microwave *Hot Bites* (Banquet)	4-½ oz	366	23	57
*****Breast, White, Canned** (Swanson)	2-½ oz	90	2	20
Breast, White and Dark, Canned:				
(Hormel)	7 oz	340	20	53
*(Swanson)	2-½ oz	100	3	27
Chunks:				
(Country Pride)	3 oz	238	15	57
Fried (Country Pride)	3 oz	276	20	65
(Tyson)	6	250	16	58
Cordon Bleu (Tyson)	5 oz	310	15	44
Croquettes (Weaver)	3-½ oz	245	15	55
Cutlets (Swanson)	3-½ oz	230	13	51
Dipsters (Swanson)	3 oz	220	14	57
Drumlets (Swanson)	3 oz	220	13	53
Frankfurter:				
(Weaver)	1	125	11	79
With Cheese (Weaver)	1	170	13	69
Fried:				
(Banquet)	6 oz	325	19	53
Hot and Spicy (Banquet)	6 oz	325	19	53
Light Crispy (Weaver)	3 oz	160	9	51
Gravy:				
Creamy (Durkee)	1 pkg	160	9	51
(Franco-American)	2 oz	50	4	72
(French's)	2 oz	25	1	51
(Heinz)	2 oz	35	2	51
Italian Hoagie (Tyson)	3 oz	250	17	61
Kiev (Tyson)	5 oz	430	31	65
Nuggets:				
(Purdue)	1 oz	73	5	62
(Weaver)	4	240	14	52
Ham and Cheese (Swanson)	3 oz	220	13	53
Hot Bites:				
(Banquet)	2-½ oz	210	14	60
Barbecue Sauce, Microwave (Banquet)	4-½ oz	360	21	52
Hot and Spicy (Banquet)	2-½ oz	246	18	66
Mexican Style (Swanson)	3 oz	220	13	53
Pizza Style (Swanson)	3 oz	210	12	51
Spinach and Herb (Swanson)	3 oz	230	13	51
Patties:				
(Country Pride)	3 oz	245	16	59
Fried (Country Pride)	3 oz	232	15	58
Rondelets (Weaver):				
Cheese	3 oz	215	13	54
Homestyle	3 oz	185	10	49

FOOD	MEASURE OR QUANTITY	CALORIES	FAT GRAMS	% FAT
Italian	3 oz	200	11	50
Original	3 oz	185	10	49
Sausage (Hormel)	4	180	16	80
Sticks:				
(Country Pride)	3 oz	233	14	54
Hot Bites (Banquet)	2-½ oz	215	15	63
Swiss 'n Bacon (Tyson)	3 oz	280	20	64
Take Out (Swanson)	3 oz	270	17	57
Tenders (Purdue)	3 oz	201	9	40
Thighs, Crispy Dutch (Weaver)	3-½ oz	295	20	61
Thighs and Drumsticks, Batter Dipped (Weaver)	3-½ oz	245	16	59
Thighs and Drumsticks, Fried (Banquet)	6 oz	245	14	51
White Roll (Weaver)	3-½ oz	130	6	42
Wings, Batter Dipped (Weaver)	3-½ oz	270	19	63
Wings, Crispy Dutch (Weaver)	3-½ oz	360	25	62
Wings, Hot & Spicy (Banquet)	4 oz	135	9	60

■ **GAME POULTRY**
Fat Range = 32% to 77%
Average Fat = 50%

FOOD	MEASURE OR QUANTITY	CALORIES	FAT GRAMS	% FAT
Duck with Skin:				
Roasted	3-½ oz	340	29	77
3-½ lb bird, Roasted	½ bird	445	25	51
Duck without Skin, Roasted	3-½ oz	200	11	50
Goose with Skin, Roasted	4 oz	350	25	64
Goose without Skin, Roasted	4 oz	270	14	47
Pheasant without Skin, Roasted	4 oz	140	5	32
Quail without Skin, Roasted	4 oz	140	5	32
Squab without Skin, Roasted	4 oz	150	8	48

■ **TURKEY PARTS**
Fat Range = 17% to 53%
Average Fat = 37%

FOOD	MEASURE OR QUANTITY	CALORIES	FAT GRAMS	% FAT
Back Half with Skin, Roasted	8-½ oz	640	38	53
Breast Half with Skin, Roasted	28 oz	1637	64	35
Dark Meat with Skin, 15-½ lb, Roasted	½ bird	1800	93	46
Dark Meat without Skin, 15-½ lb., Roasted	½ bird	1300	51	35

FOOD	MEASURE OR QUANTITY	CALORIES	FAT GRAMS	% FAT
Leg, Roasted	18 oz	1200	55	41
Light & Dark Meat with Skin, Roasted	3½ oz	200	10	45
***Light and Dark Meat without Skin,** Roasted	3-½ oz	170	5	26
***Light Meat without Skin,** Roasted	3-½ oz	160	3	17
***Light Meat without Skin 15-½ lb.,** Roasted	½ bird	1400	30	19
Light Meat with Skin, Roasted	3-½ oz	200	8	36
Light Meat with Skin, 15-½ lb., Roasted	½ bird	2070	87	38
Meat with Skin, Roasted	3-½ oz	208	10	43
***Meat without Skin,** Roasted	3-½ oz	170	5	26
Wing with Skin, Roasted	6 oz	430	23	48

■ TURKEY, PROCESSED
Fat Range = 0% to 81%
Average Fat = 40%

FOOD	MEASURE OR QUANTITY	CALORIES	FAT GRAMS	% FAT
Bologna, Turkey (Louis Rich)	1 slice	58	5	78
Breast:				
*(Land O' Lakes)	3 oz	100	1	9
*(Louis Rich)	1 slice	44	1	20
(Louis Rich)	1 oz	50	2	36
*(Oscar Meyer)	1 slice	20	0	0
(Weaver)	3 oz	105	4	34
***Breast, Barbecue** (Louis Rich)	1 oz	40	1	22
Breast, Broth Baste (Land O' Lakes)	3 oz	120	5	38
Breast, Butter Baste (Land O' Lakes)	3 oz	140	8	51
***Breast Roll** (Weaver)	3 oz	100	1	9
Breast Roll, White Meat:				
Blue (Land O' Lakes)	3 oz	110	5	41
Red (Land O' Lakes)	3 oz	110	5	41
Breast Roll, White and Dark:				
Blue (Land O' Lakes)	3 oz	110	5	41
Red (Land O' Lakes)	3 oz	120	6	45
***Breast, Smoked** (Louis Rich)	1 slice	33	1	27
***Breast with Skin** (Boar's Head)	1 oz	40	1	22
***Breast without Skin** (Boar's Head)	1 oz	32	0	0
Frankfurter:				
(Armour Star)	1	110	8	65
Cheese (Louis Rich)	1	108	9	75
(Louis Rich)	1	100	9	81
Gravy:				
(Franco-American)	2 oz	30	2	60

FOOD	MEASURE OR QUANTITY	CALORIES	FAT GRAMS	% FAT
(French's)	2 fl oz	25	1	36
Homestyle (Heinz)	2 oz	30	2	60
Ham:				
*(Louis Rich)	1 slice	35	1	26
(Weaver)	1 oz	140	6	39
Luncheon Loaf (Louis Rich)	1 slice	40	2	45
Meat Loaf (Armour)	3 oz	160	8	45
Pastrami:				
(Armour)	4 oz	140	5	32
*(Louis Rich)	1 slice	35	1	26
Salami (Louis Rich)	1 slice	60	4	60
Sausage:				
(Louis Rich)	1 oz	65	4	55
Smoked (Louis Rich)	1	55	4	65

26. SANDWICHES AND SIDE DISHES

■ SANDWICHES

SANDWICHES ARE MADE WITH 4 OZ OF FILLER AND 2 SLICES OF BREAD

Fat Range = 20% to 73%
Average Fat = 51%

FOOD	MEASURE OR QUANTITY	CALORIES	FAT GRAMS	% FAT
Bologna	1	480	34	64
BLT (3 Sl Bacon) with				
Mayonnaise	1	420	21	45
Cheese Sandwich, American				
Cheese	1	550	40	65
Chicken, Fried	1	540	28	47
Chicken Breast, Grilled:				
With Mayonnaise	1	440	17	35
*Without Mayonnaise	1	330	11	30
Corned Beef, 6 Ounces	1	800	60	68
Egg Salad	1	570	42	66
Egg, Sliced	1	340	19	50
Fish, Fried	1	545	30	50
Grilled Cheese:				
And Bacon	1	680	44	58
And Tomato	1	600	36	54

FOOD	MEASURE OR QUANTITY	CALORIES	FAT GRAMS	% FAT
Ham Sandwich:				
And Cheese	1	540	35	58
Plain	1	420	22	47
Hamburger	1	650	40	55
Hot Dog, on Roll	1	340	18	48
Liverwurst	1	550	34	56
Pastrami, 6 Ounces	1	660	53	72
Peanut Butter and Jelly, 3 Tablespoons Peanut Butter	1	560	25	40
Reuben	1	1300	75	52
Roast Beef:				
And Cheese	1	660	41	56
Plain	1	660	33	45
Salami	1	480	34	64
Shrimp Salad	1	500	30	54
Tuna Melt and Cheese	1	900	49	49
Tuna Salad	1	770	40	47
Turkey Breast:				
With Mayonnaise	1	420	18	39
*Without Mayonnaise	1	380	7	20
Turkey Club, with Bacon and Tomato				
With Mayonnaise	1	850	34	36
*Without Mayonnaise	1	750	23	25
Turkey Salad	1	580	35	54

■ SANDWICH SIDE DISHES

Fat Range = 0% to 99%
Average Fat = 68%

FOOD	MEASURE OR QUANTITY	CALORIES	FAT GRAMS	% FAT
Butter	1 T	100	11	99
Cole Slaw	1 T	20	2	90
Cole Slaw	4 oz	70	7	90
French Fries	1 serv	250	14	50
*Ketchup	1 T	15	0	0
Margarine	1 T	100	11	99
Mayonnaise:				
Light	1 T	50	5	90
Regular	1 T	100	11	99
*Mustard	1 T	15	0	0
Potato Salad	2 T	40	3	68
Potato Salad	4 oz	160	12	68

27. SNACK AND JUNK FOOD

■ CANDY

Fat Range = 0% to 72%
Average Fat = 34%

FOOD	MEASURE OR QUANTITY	CALORIES	FAT GRAMS	% FAT
Almond Joy	1.6 oz	220	12	49
Baby Ruth	1 oz	130	6	42
Bit-O-Honey	1.7 oz	200	4	18
Bonkers!	1 piece	20	0	0
Bridge Mix	1 oz	130	5	35
Butterfinger	1 bar	260	12	42
Cadbury's (Peter Paul):				
Chocolate Almond	2 oz	310	18	52
Cream Eggs	1 item	200	7	32
Eggs, Small	1 oz	140	7	45
Fruit Nut Bar	2 oz	300	16	48
Hazelnut Chocolate	2 oz	310	17	49
Milk Chocolate	2 oz	300	16	48
Coffioca Parfait (Pearson)	4 pieces	120	2	22
Candy Corn	20 pieces	180	0	0
Caramel (Kraft)	1 piece	35	1	26
Caramel Nip (Pearson)	2 pieces	60	1	15
Caramello Bar	2 oz	280	13	42
Charleston Chew!	½ bar	120	3	22
Chocolate Covered Cherries	1 piece	120	4	30
Chocolate Covered Peanuts	15 pieces	160	9	51
Chocolate Covered Raisins	30 pieces	120	4	30
Chocolate Fudgies	1 piece	35	1	26
Chocolate Parfait (Pearson)	2 pieces	60	1	15
Chuckles, All Flavors	1 oz	100	0	0
Clark Bar	1 oz	134	5	34
Coffee Nip (Pearson)	2 pieces	60	1	15
Coffioca Parfait	2 pieces	60	1	15
Good & Fruity	1 oz	105	0	0
Good & Plenty	1 oz	105	0	0
Gummy Bears	4 pieces	20	0	0
Halvah	1 oz	150	10	60
Hershey's:				
Almond Chocolate Bar	1-½ oz	230	14	55
Chocolate Bar	1-½ oz	220	13	53
Golden Almond Bar	1 oz	160	11	62
Kisses	6 pieces	150	9	54
Special Dark	1-½ oz	220	12	49
Jelly Beans	10 pieces	200	0	0
Junior Mints	12 pieces	120	3	22
KitKat	1-½ oz	210	11	47
Krackel	1-½ oz	220	12	49

FOOD	MEASURE OR QUANTITY	CALORIES	FAT GRAMS	% FAT
*Licorice Nip (Pearsons)	2 pieces	60	1	15
M&M's				
Peanut	1.7 oz	250	13	47
Plain	1.7 oz	240	10	38
Mallo Cups (Boyer)	2	224	11	44
Malted Milk Balls	4 pieces	100	8	72
Mars	1 bar	240	11	41
Marshmallow:				
*Large	2 pieces	40	0	0
*Small	24 pieces	40	0	0
*Milk Shake	2 oz	250	8	29
Milky Way	2 oz	270	10	33
Mounds	1.7 oz	230	12	47
Mr. Goodbar	1.7 oz	250	15	54
Necco Sky Bar	1 bar	176	8	41
Nestlé:				
Crunch	1.2 oz	160	8	45
Almond Milk Chocolate	1 oz	160	10	56
Milk Chocolate	1 oz	150	9	54
White Almond	1 oz	170	12	64
Park Avenue	1 bar	230	9	35
Pay Day	1 bar	250	12	43
Peanut Bar (Planters)	1.5 oz	230	13	51
*Peanut Brittle	1 oz	120	3	22
*Peanut Butter Parfait (Pearson)	4 pieces	120	3	22
Peanut Cluster	1 oz	150	9	54
*Pom Poms Caramel	1 oz	100	3	27
PowerHouse	2.2 oz	290	11	34
Reese's Peanut Butter Cups:				
Crunchy	2 cups	240	14	52
Plain	2 cups	240	14	52
Reese's Pieces	30 pieces	130	5	35
Rolo	5 pieces	140	6	39
*Skittles	2 oz	320	5	14
Snickers	2.2 oz	290	14	43
*Starburst	2 oz	240	5	19
Symphony (Hershey's):				
Almond Toffee Bar	1 bar	220	14	57
Chocolate Bar	1 bar	180	13	65
*Thin Mint	1 item	40	1	22
*3 Musketeers	2 oz	250	8	29
*Tootsie Roll	1 small	25	0	0
Twix:				
Peanut	2 pieces	130	7	48
Plain	2 pieces	140	7	45
*Twizzlers	1 oz	100	0	0
*Valentine Sugar Heart	1 piece	5	0	0
Whatchamacallit	1.5 oz	210	12	51
*Yogurt Covered Raisins	1 oz	120	3	22
*York Peppermint Patty	1 patty	180	5	25
*Zagnut	1 oz	130	4	28
Zero	1 bar	250	10	36

■ **CORN CHIPS**
Fat Range = 30% to 73%
Average Fat = 73%

FOOD	MEASURE OR QUANTITY	CALORIES	FAT GRAMS	% FAT
Bachman:				
BBQ	1 oz	150	9	54
Plain	1 oz	150	9	54
Nacho	1 oz	140	6	39
Tortilla	1 oz	140	8	51
Bugles	1 oz	150	8	48
Cheez Balls (Planters)	1 oz	160	10	56
Chee-Tos	1 oz	160	10	56
Cheese 'n Crunch	1 oz	160	11	62
Cheez Doodles:				
Crunchy	1 oz	160	10	56
Regular	1 oz	160	10	56
Corn Chip (Store Brand)	1 oz	150	9	54
Corn Crunchies (Wise)	1 oz	160	10	56
Cornnuts	1 oz	120	4	30
Dipsy Doodles (Wise)	1 oz	160	10	56
Doo-Dads	1 oz	140	6	39
Doritos:				
Cool Ranch	1 oz	140	7	45
Regular	1 oz	140	7	45
Nacho Cheese Flavor	1 oz	140	7	45
Taco	1 oz	140	7	45
Tortilla Chips, Salsa	1 oz	140	7	45
Eagle	1 oz	150	8	48
Frito's (Frito-Lay):				
BBQ	1 oz	150	9	54
Plain	1 oz	150	9	54
Jax:				
Crunchy	1 oz	160	11	62
Plain	1 oz	150	8	48
Planters:				
Plain	1 oz	160	10	56
Tortilla	1 oz	150	8	48
Tom's:				
BBQ	1 oz	160	13	73
Plain	1 oz	150	8	48
Tortilla	1 oz	200	7	32
Tortilla Nachos (Lance)	1 oz	150	8	48

■ **DIPS**
Fat Range = 60% to 80%
Average Fat = 69%

FOOD	MEASURE OR QUANTITY	CALORIES	FAT GRAMS	% FAT
Avocado, Guacamole (Kraft)	2 T	50	4	72
Bacon and Horseradish (Kraft)	2 T	60	5	75

FOOD	MEASURE OR QUANTITY	CALORIES	FAT GRAMS	% FAT
Blue Cheese (Kraft)	2 T	45	4	80
Clam (Kraft)	2 T	60	4	60
Garlic (Kraft)	2 T	60	4	60
Jalapeño Pepper (Kraft)	2 T	50	4	72
Nacho Cheese (Kraft)	2 T	50	4	72
Onion, Creamy (Kraft)	2 T	45	4	80
Onion, French (Kraft)	2 T	60	4	60
Onion, Green (Kraft)	2 T	60	4	60

■ GRANOLA BARS
Fat Range = 18% to 54%
Average = 36%

FOOD	MEASURE OR QUANTITY	CALORIES	FAT GRAMS	% FAT
*Almond Clusters (Nature Valley)	1	150	4	24
Almond, Roasted (Nature Valley)	1	120	5	38
Apple, Chewy (Nature Valley)	1	130	5	35
*Apple Clusters (Nature Valley)	1	150	4	24
*Caramel Clusters (Nature Valley)	1	150	3	18
Caramel Nut (*Dipps*)	1	150	6	36
Chocolate Chip:				
Chewy (Nature Valley)	1	150	7	42
*Clusters (Nature Valley)	1	150	4	24
Dipps (Quaker)	1	140	6	39
(Kudos)	1	180	9	45
(New Trail)	1	190	9	43
*Chocolate Clusters (Nature Valley)	1	140	3	19
Chocolate Covered:				
Honey (New Trail)	1	200	12	54
Peanut Butter (New Trail)	1	200	11	50
Chunky Nut and Raisin, *Dipps*				
(Quaker)	1	130	6	42
Cinnamon (Nature Valley)	1	110	4	33
Cinnamon Raisin (Quaker)	1	130	5	35
*Fruit and Apple (Nature Valley)	1	150	5	30
*Fruit and Date (Nature Valley)	1	160	5	28
Honey and Oats:				
*(Quaker)	1	130	4	28
Dipps (Quaker)	1	140	6	39
(Nature Valley)	1	110	4	33
Mint Chocolate Chip *Dipps*				
(Quaker)	1	140	6	39
Nutty Fudge (Kudos)	1	190	11	52
Peanut (Nature Valley)	1	120	5	38
Peanut Butter:				
Chewy (Nature Valley)	1	140	6	39
Dipps (Quaker)	1	150	7	42
(Kudos)	1	190	11	52
(Nature Valley)	1	120	6	45
(New Trail)	1	190	9	43
(Quaker)	1	140	6	39

FOOD	MEASURE OR QUANTITY	CALORIES	FAT GRAMS	% FAT
Peanut Butter and Chocolate Chips				
(Quaker)	1	130	5	35
Raisin and Almond Dipps				
(Quaker)	1	140	6	39
Raisin, Chewy (Nature Valley)	1	130	5	35
***Raisin Cluster** (Nature Valley)	1	150	3	18
Rocky Road *Dipps* (Quaker)	1	140	7	45

■ GUM AND HARD CANDY
Fat Range = 0% to 15%
Average Fat = 15%

FOOD	MEASURE OR QUANTITY	CALORIES	FAT GRAMS	% FAT
***Beech-Nut Gum, All Flavors**	1 stick	10	0	0
***Breath Savers**	1	8	0	0
Bubble Yum				
*All Flavors	1 stick	25	0	0
*Sugarless, All Flavors	1 stick	20	0	0
***Canada Mint**	1 piece	12	0	0
Care*Free				
*Bubble Gum, All Flavors	1 stick	10	0	0
*Gum, All Flavors	1 stick	8	0	0
***Cin-O-Mon,** *Wint-O-Green*				
Lifesavers	1	7	0	0
***Cough Drop, All Flavors**	1	10	0	0
***Extra Sugar Free**	1 stick	8	0	0
***Freedent**, All Flavors	1 stick	10	0	0
***Gum Drops**	1 oz	90	1	10
***Hubba-Bubba**, All Flavors	1 stick	23	0	0
***Juicy Fruit**	1 stick	10	0	0
***Lifesaver**, All Flavors	1	10	0	0
***Lollipops, All Flavors**				
(Lifesavers)	1	45	0	0
***Skittles**	1 oz	115	1	8
***Sour Ball, Hard**	2	25	0	0
***Starburst**	1 oz	120	2	15
***Sugar Daddy**	1	150	1	6
***Tic Tac**	1	1	0	0
***Tootsie Pop**, All Flavors	1	110	0	0

■ POPCORN
Fat Range = 0% to 77%
Average Fat = 42%

FOOD	MEASURE OR QUANTITY	CALORIES	FAT GRAMS	% FAT
Air Popped:				
*Homemade	1 cup	25	0	0
*Homemade	4 cups	100	0	0
White Cheddar (Bachman)	1 oz	70	4	51
Bachman	4 cups	160	11	62
*_Cracker Jack_	4 cups	120	3	22
Jiffy-Pop Pan	4 cups	130	6	42
Lance, Cheese	1 pkg	130	8	55
Lite Cheddar Gourmet (Boston Popcorn)	1 oz	70	4	51
Lite Handcooked Gourmet (Boston Popcorn)	1 oz	60	3	45
Microwave:				
*Dry Kernels—No Oil Homemade	1 cup	25	0	0
*Homemade	1 cup	25	0	0
*Homemade	4 cups	100	0	0
(Jiffy Pop)	4 cups	140	7	45
(Jolly Time)	3 cups	150	8	48
(Newman's Own)	3 cups	150	8	48
(Pillsbury)	4 cups	260	15	52
(Pop Rite)	4 cups	167	7	38
(T.V. Time)	4 cups	230	14	55
Microwave, Butter:				
*(Orville Redenbacher's)	4 cups	260	7	24
(Pop Secret)	4 cups	230	13	51
Microwave, Caramel (Orville Redenbacher's)	2-½ cups	240	14	52
Microwave, Cheddar (Orville Redenbacher's)	3 cups	150	10	60
Microwave, Cheese (Pop Secret)	3 cups	170	11	58
Microwave, Light:				
*(Orville Redenbacher's)	3 cups	60	2	30
(Pop Secret)	3 cups	70	3	39
Microwave, No Salt (Orville Redenbacher's)	3 cups	90	6	60
Microwave, Original:				
(Orville Redenbacher's)	4 cups	140	8	51
(Planters)	3 cups	140	10	64
Popped with Oil:				
Homemade	1 cup	55	3	49
*Regular (Orville Redenbacher's)	4 cups	90	1	10
Smartfood	1 oz	160	10	56
*White Jolly Time Oil	4 cups	75	1	12
Wise:				
Butter Popped	1 oz	80	5	56
Tender Eating	2 cups	70	6	77

FOOD	MEASURE OR QUANTITY	CALORIES	FAT GRAMS	% FAT
With Cheese	½ oz	90	6	60
With White Cheese	2 cups	70	5	64

■ POTATO CHIPS
Fat Range = 38% to 71%
Average Fat = 71%

FOOD	MEASURE OR QUANTITY	CALORIES	FAT GRAMS	% FAT
Bachman:				
BBQ	1 oz	150	9	54
Hot	1 oz	150	9	54
Regular	1 oz	160	10	56
Sour Cream and Onion	1 oz	150	9	54
Cape Cod	1 oz	150	8	48
Charles' Chips:				
Bacon and Cheese	1 oz	160	10	56
Hot Jalapeño	1 oz	160	10	56
No Salt	1 oz	160	10	56
Original	1 oz	160	10	56
Chipsters	1 oz	120	5	38
Cottage Fries	1 oz	160	11	62
Eagle	1 oz	150	10	60
Generic	1 oz	160	10	56
Health Valley	1 oz	160	10	56
Krunchers:				
Alfredo	1 oz	150	9	54
Jalapeño	1 oz	150	9	54
Original	1 oz	150	9	54
Lance:				
Original	1-⅛ oz	190	15	71
Sour Cream and Onion	1-⅛ oz	190	12	57
Lays:				
Original	1-⅛ oz	170	11	58
Salt and Vinegar	1 oz	150	9	54
New York Deli	1 oz	160	11	62
Pringles:				
Light	1 oz	150	8	48
Regular	1 oz	170	13	69
Rippled	1 oz	170	12	64
Sour Cream and Onion	1 oz	170	12	64
Ruffles:				
Bacon and Sour Cream	1 oz	160	10	56
Original	1 oz	150	10	60
Sour Cream and Onion	1 oz	150	9	54
Suncher, Ranch Chips	1 oz	150	8	48
Wise, Regular	1 oz	160	11	62

■ PRETZELS
Fat Range = 0% to 17%
Average Fat = 17%

FOOD	MEASURE OR QUANTITY	CALORIES	FAT GRAMS	% FAT
*(Anderson) *Bavarian Baldies*	1 oz	110	1	8
Bachmann:				
*Hard	1 oz	102	0	0
*Rods	1 rod	110	2	16
*Eagle	1 oz	110	1	8
Lance:				
*Regular	1 oz	100	1	9
*Twist	1-½ oz	150	1	6
Mister Salty:				
*Dutch	2	110	1	8
*Mini Mix	1 oz	110	1	8
*Nuggets	21 pieces	110	1	8
*Rings	25	115	2	16
*Sticks	90 pieces	110	1	8
*Veri-Thin	45 pieces	110	1	8
*Pretzel (Store Brand)	1 oz	110	1	8
Quinlan:				
*Beer	1 oz	110	1	8
*Cheese Thins	1 oz	109	2	17
*Logs	1 oz	110	2	16
*Tiny Thins	1 oz	108	1	8
Reisman:				
*Hard	1 oz	107	1	8
*Mini	1 oz	110	1	8
*Thin Sticks	1 oz	110	1	8
Snyder's:				
*Hard	1 oz	102	0	0
*Thins	1 oz	110	2	16

28. SOUPS

■ SOUPS
Fat Range = 0% to 77%
Average Fat = 28%

FOOD	MEASURE OR QUANTITY	CALORIES	FAT GRAMS	% FAT
Asparagus, Cream of (Campbell's)	1 cup	90	4	40
*Bacon Bean	1 cup	178	6	30

FOOD	MEASURE OR QUANTITY	CALORIES	FAT GRAMS	% FAT
Bean and Ham:				
*(Campbell's)	10 fl oz	260	8	28
*(Progresso)	9 fl oz	170	1	5
Beef:				
*(Campbell's)	1 cup	80	2	22
*Chunky (Campbell's)	10 fl oz	170	4	21
Beef Bouillon Cube:				
*(Herb-Ox)	1	6	0	0
*(Wyler's)	1	10	0	0
*Beef Broth	1 cup	12	0	0
*Beef Broth	1 cube	8	0	0
Beef Broth and Seasoning:				
*(Weight Watchers)	1 pkg	10	0	0
*Cup-A-Soup (Lipton)	7 fl oz	120	2	15
Beef, Ham:				
*Chunky (Campbell's)	11 fl oz	290	9	28
*(Progresso)	10 fl oz	170	1	5
*Beef Minestrone (Progresso)	9 fl oz	150	4	24
Beef Noodle:				
(Campbell's)	1 cup	70	3	39
Homestyle (Campbell's)	1 cup	90	4	40
*(Lipton)	6 fl oz	45	1	20
Beef Vegetable Noodle:				
*(Campbell's)	1 cup	80	1	11
*(Lipton) Cup-A-Soup	1 cup	80	1	11
Black Bean:				
*(Campbell's)	1 cup	110	2	16
*(Progresso)	1 cup	122	2	15
*Borscht, Low Calorie				
(Manischewitz)	1 cup	20	0	0
*Borscht, Regular (Rokeach)	1 cup	100	1	9
Celery, Cream of:				
(Campbell's)	1 cup	100	7	63
(Rokeach)	10 fl oz	90	4	40
Cheddar Cheese (Campbell's)	1 cup	130	8	55
Cheese in Milk (Campbell's)	1 cup	226	14	56
Chicken Alphabet (Campbell's)	1 cup	80	3	34
Chicken Broth:				
*(Homemade)	1 cup	33	1	27
*(Pritikin)	7 fl oz	60	1	15
Chicken, Chunky (Campbell's)	1 cup	183	7	34
Chicken, Cream of:				
(Campbell's)	1 cup	110	7	57
In Milk (Campbell's)	1 cup	196	12	55
(Lipton)	6 fl oz	80	4	45
*With Noodle (Campbell's)	6 fl oz	150	5	30
Chicken Dumplings:				
(Lipton)	1 cup	102	6	53
(Campbell's)	1 cup	80	3	34
*Chicken Gumbo (Campbell's)	1 cup	60	2	30
*Chicken Hearty (Campbell's)	6 fl oz	70	1	13
*Chicken Meat with Noodles				
(Campbell's)	6 fl oz	45	1	20
Chicken Minestrone (Progresso)	9 fl oz	150	6	36
Chicken Noodle:				
*(Campbell's)	1 cup	70	2	26

FOOD	MEASURE OR QUANTITY	CALORIES	FAT GRAMS	% FAT
Dehydrated Package (Knorr)	1 cup	58	2	31
*(Lipton)	1 cup	70	2	26
*(Store Brand)	1 cup	70	2	26
Chicken Rice:				
*(Campbell's)	1 cup	127	3	21
*(Lipton)	6 fl oz	45	1	20
*Chicken Stars (Campbell's)	1 cup	60	2	30
*Chicken, Steak and Potato				
(Lipton)	1 cup	200	5	22
Chicken Supreme (Lipton)	6 fl oz	100	5	45
Chicken Vegetable				
(Campbell's)	1 cup	70	3	39
Chili Beef:				
(Campbell's)	1 cup	175	7	36
*Chunk (Campbell's)	11 fl oz	290	7	22
Clam Chowder, Manhattan Style:				
*(Campbell's)	1 cup	70	2	26
*(Doxee)	6 fl oz	50	0	0
Clam Chowder, New England Style:				
(Campbell's)	1 cup	80	3	34
(Stouffer's)	1 cup	200	10	45
With Milk (Campbell's)	11 fl oz	200	8	36
*Consomme (Campbell's)	1 cup	28	0	0
Corn Chowder with Milk				
(Snow's)	1 cup	150	6	36
*Crab Soup (Campbell's)	1 cup	78	2	23
Escarole:				
In Chicken Broth (Progresso)	9 fl oz	35	3	77
(Progresso)	1 cup	34	2	53
Fish Chowder (Snow's)	1 cup	140	6	39
French Onion (Progresso)	9 fl oz	120	9	68
Gazpacho (Progresso)	1 cup	58	2	31
Green Pea:				
(Campbell's)	1 cup	100	4	36
*Lipton	6 fl oz	120	4	30
*With Milk (Campbell's)	1 cup	239	7	26
Ham & Butter Bean (Campbell's)	6 fl oz	280	10	32
Lentil				
*(Progresso)	9 fl oz	170	2	11
*With Ham (Progresso)	1 cup	143	3	19
Meatball Alphabet (Campbell's)	1 cup	100	4	36
Minestrone:				
(Campbell's)	1 cup	87	3	31
*(Progresso)	9 fl oz	160	4	22
Minestrone and Beef				
(Campbell's)	1 cup	60	3	45
*Minestrone, Cream (Campbell's)	4 fl oz	80	2	22
Mushroom, Cream of:				
(Campbell's)	1 cup	100	7	63
(Lipton)	6 fl oz	80	4	45
*Noodle Giggle (Lipton)	1 cup	80	2	22
Onion:				
*(Campbell's)	1 cup	66	2	27
*Dehydrated Pakage (Knorr)	1 pkg	118	2	15
Oyster Stew (Campbell's)	1 cup	132	8	55

FOOD	MEASURE OR QUANTITY	CALORIES	FAT GRAMS	% FAT
Potato, Cream of (Campbell's)	1 cup	146	6	37
Seafood Chowder, New England Style (Snow's)	1 cup	130	6	42
Shrimp, Cream of (Campbell's)	1 cup	161	9	50
Split Pea:				
*(Store Brand)	1 cup	188	4	19
*(Stouffer's)	1 cup	185	3	15
*Split Pea with Ham (Campbell's)	1 cup	170	4	21
*Tomato (Campbell's)	1 cup	90	2	20
*Tomato Beef Noodle (Campbell's)	1 cup	136	4	26
Tomato Bisque:				
*(Campbell's)	1 cup	120	3	22
With Milk (Campbell's)	1 cup	203	7	31
Tomato, Cream of (Campbell's)	1 cup	166	6	33
*Tomato Consomme Cup-A-Soup (Lipton)	6 fl oz	80	1	11
*Tomato Onion (Lipton)	1 cup	70	1	13
*Tomato Rice (Campbell's)	1 cup	110	2	16
*Tomato Vegetable Cup-A-Soup (Lipton)	7 fl oz	110	1	8
*Turkey Noodle (Campbell's)	1 cup	66	2	27
Turkey Vegetable (Campbell's)	1 cup	70	3	39
Vegetable:				
(Campbell's)	1 cup	70	3	39
*(Lipton)	1 cup	80	1	11
Vegetable Beef:				
*(Campbell's)	1 cup	78	2	23
*Chunky (Campbell's)	10 fl oz	180	5	25
Vegetable, Bouillon Cube				
*(Herb Ox)	1	6	0	0
*Garden (Lipton)	7 fl oz	130	2	14
*Mediterranean (Campbell's)	4 fl oz	160	5	28
*Spanish (Campbell's)	1 cup	40	0	0
*In Water (Campbell's)	1 cup	74	2	24
Vichyssoise (Campbell's)	1 cup	146	6	37
*Won Ton (Campbell's)	1 cup	40	1	22

29. STAPLES

■ JELLIES, JAMS, AND PRESERVES
Fat Range = 0%
Average Fat = 0%

FOOD	MEASURE OR QUANTITY	CALORIES	FAT GRAMS	% FAT
Apple Butter:				
*(Smucker's)	1 T	36	0	0
*(Smucker's)	1 t	12	0	0
*Honey (Store Brand)	1 T	65	0	0
*Jam (Store Brand)	1 packet	40	0	0
Jelly, All Flavors:				
*(Kraft)	1 T	48	0	0
*(Kraft)	1 t	16	0	0
*(Pritikin)	1 T	42	0	0
*(Pritikin)	1 t	14	0	0
*(Smucker's)	1 T	48	0	0
*(Smucker's)	1 t	16	0	0
*(Store Brand)	1 packet	40	0	0
*(Welch's)	1 T	48	0	0
*(Welch's)	1 t	16	0	0
Jelly, All Flavors, Low Sugar:				
*(Smucker's)	1 T	24	0	0
*(Smucker's)	1 t	8	0	0
Preserves, All Flavors:				
*(Estee)	1 T	6	0	0
*(Estee)	1 t	2	0	0
*(Kraft)	1 T	48	0	0
*(Kraft)	1 t	16	0	0

■ SUGAR AND SUGAR SUSTITUTES
Fat Range = 0%
Average Fat = 0%

FOOD	MEASURE OR QUANTITY	CALORIES	FAT GRAMS	% FAT
Brown Sugar:				
*Not Packed	1 cup	550	0	0
*Packed	1 cup	830	0	0
*Equal	1 envlp	4	0	0
*Equal	1 t	0	0	0
*Sweet 'n Low	1 envlp	4	0	0
*Sweet 'n Low	1 t	0	0	0
*White Sugar Granulated	1 cup	770	0	0
*White Sugar Granulated	1 t	15	0	0
*White Sugar Granulated	1 T	50	0	0

FOOD	MEASURE OR QUANTITY	CALORIES	FAT GRAMS	% FAT
*Honey	1 t	22	0	0
*Honey	1 T	65	0	0

■ SYRUPS
Fat Range = 0%
Average Fat = 0%

FOOD	MEASURE OR QUANTITY	CALORIES	FAT GRAMS	% FAT
(Aunt Jemima):				
*Butter Lite	1 T	30	0	0
*Regular	1 T	50	0	0
Corn:				
*(Karo)	1 T	60	0	0
*Light (Karo)	1 T	60	0	0
*Regular	1 T	60	0	0
*Golden Griddle	1 T	60	0	0
Log Cabin:				
*Buttered	1 T	51	0	0
*Country Kitchen	1 T	50	0	0
*Lite	1 T	30	0	0
*Maple Honey	1 T	50	0	0
*Regular	1 T	50	0	0
*Maple Syrup, Vermont	1 T	50	0	0
*Molasses Cane, Vermont	1 T	50	0	0
Mrs. Butterworth's:				
*Lite	1 T	30	0	0
*Regular	1 T	55	0	0

30. STARCH

■ FLOUR AND GRAINS
Fat Range = 0% to 44%
Average Fat = 7%

FOOD	MEASURE OR QUANTITY	CALORIES	FAT GRAMS	% FAT
Barley, Medium:				
*(Quaker Scotch)	¼ cup	170	0	0
*(Scotch)	1 cup	700	2	3

FOOD	MEASURE OR QUANTITY	CALORIES	FAT GRAMS	% FAT
*Barley, Pearled, Light	1 cup	700	2	3
Buckwheat Flour:				
*Dark	1 cup	330	3	8
*Light	1 cup	340	1	3
*Bisquick (General Mills)	2 oz	240	8	30
*Carob Flour	1 cup	185	1	5
*Corn Flour	1 cup	430	3	6
Corn Meal Mix:				
*Buttermilk (Aunt Jemina)	1 oz	100	1	9
*White Bolted (Aunt Jemina)	1/6 cup	100	1	9
Corn Meal, White:				
*Bolted	1 cup	440	4	8
*Degermed	1 cup	500	2	4
*Degermed (Aunt Jemina)	1 oz	100	1	9
Corn Meal, Yellow:				
*Bolted	1 cup	500	2	4
*Degermed	1 cup	500	2	4
*Whole Ground	1 cup	430	5	10
*Millet, Whole Grain	4 oz	330	3	8
*Oat Bran (Quaker)	1 cup	330	7	19
*Peanut Flour	1 cup	200	1	4
*Potato Flour	1 cup	640	2	3
*Rye Flour	1 cup	420	3	6
*Softasilk (General Mills)	1 cup	400	1	2
*Sorghum Grain	4 oz	340	4	11
*Soy Meal, No Fat	1 cup	411	3	7
Soybean Flour:				
Full Fat	1 cup	370	18	44
*Low Fat	1 cup	330	6	16
*No Fat	1 cup	330	1	3
*St. Johnsbread Flour	1 cup	185	1	5
Wheat Bran:				
*(Kretchmer)	1 oz	60	1	15
*Wheat Bran (Quaker)	2 T	20	0	0
Wheat Flour:				
*All Purpose (Pillsbury)	1 cup	400	1	2
*Bread (Pillsbury)	1 cup	400	3	7
*Cake (Pillsbury)	1 cup	430	1	2
*High Protein (Gold Medal)	1 cup	400	1	2
*(La Pina)	1 cup	400	1	2
*Regular	1 cup	500	1	2
*Self Rising (Ballard)	1 cup	400	1	2
*Self Rising (Gold Medal)	1 cup	400	1	2
*Unbleached (Pillsbury)	1 cup	400	2	4
*Whole (Pillsbury)	1 cup	400	2	4
*Wheat, White (Ballard)	1 cup	400	1	2
*White (Wondra)	1 cup	400	1	2

■ PASTA DISHES, CANNED
Fat Range = 6% to 42%
Average Fat = 26%

FOOD	MEASURE OR QUANTITY	CALORIES	FAT GRAMS	% FAT
ABC's & 123's:				
*(Chef Boyardee)	7-½ oz	160	1	6
And Meatballs (Chef Boyardee)	7-½ oz	240	9	34
Beef-O-Getti (Chef Boyardee)	7-½ oz	220	9	37
Beef Ravioli:				
*(Chef Boyardee)	7-½ oz	180	5	25
*And Sauce (Chef Boyardee)	7-½ oz	240	6	22
Beefaroni (Chef Boyardee)	7-½ oz	220	8	33
Cheese Ravioli:				
*And Beef (Chef Boyardee)	7-½ oz	200	3	14
*Tomato (Chef Boyardee)	7-½ oz	200	5	22
***Chicken Ravioli** (Chef Boyardee)	7-½ oz	180	4	20
Dinosaurs:				
*Chef Boyardee	7-½ oz	155	1	6
And Meatballs (Chef Boyardee)	7-½ oz	235	8	31
Lasagna (Chef Boyardee)	7-½ oz	230	8	31
Macaroni and Beef:				
(Franco-American)	7-½ oz	220	8	33
(Heinz)	7-½ oz	200	8	36
Macaroni and Cheese:				
*(Franco-American)	7-½ oz	170	5	26
(Heinz)	7-½ oz	190	8	38
***Macaroni and Shells**				
(Chef Boyardee)	7-½ oz	150	1	6
Macaroni, Elbows and Cheese				
(Franco-American)	7-½ oz	170	6	32
***Mini Beef Ravioli**				
(Chef Boyardee)	7-½ oz	210	5	21
Mini Bites (Chef Boyardee)	7-½ oz	260	12	42
***Mini Canneloni** (Chef Boyardee)	7-½ oz	230	7	27
Mini Chicken Ravioli				
(Chef Boyardee)	7-½ oz	220	8	33
Pac-Man (Chef Boyardee)				
Chicken	7-½ oz	170	7	37
Meatballs	7-½ oz	230	9	35
*Tomato	7-½ oz	150	1	6
***RavioliOs** (Franco-American)	7-½ oz	210	5	21
Roller Coasters (Chef Boyardee)	7-½ oz	230	9	35
Smurf (Chef Boyardee):				
*Beef Ravioli	7-½ oz	220	5	20
*Beef Spaghetti	7-½ oz	150	1	6
Meatballs	7-½ oz	230	9	35
Spaghetti & Franks				
(Franco-American)	7-½ oz	220	9	37
Spaghetti and Meatballs:				
(Chef Boyardee)	7-½ oz	230	8	31
(Franco-American)	7-½ oz	220	8	33
Spaghetti in Meat Sauce				
(Franco-American)	7-½ oz	210	8	34
Spaghetti, Tomato and Cheese				
*(Heinz)	7-½ oz	160	2	11

FOOD	MEASURE OR QUANTITY	CALORIES	FAT GRAMS	% FAT
Tic Tac Toes:				
And Meatballs (Chef Boyardee)	7-½ oz	240	9	34
*Spaghetti (Chef Boyardee)	7-½ oz	160	1	6
UFO's:				
*(Franco-American)	7-½ oz	180	3	15
With Meteors				
(Franco-American)	7-½ oz	230	8	31
***Zooroni and Meatballs**				
(Chef Boyardee)	7-½ oz	240	8	30

■ PASTA DISHES, FROZEN
Fat Range = 12% to 60%
Average Fat = 33%

FOOD	MEASURE OR QUANTITY	CALORIES	FAT GRAMS	% FAT
Cheese Ravioli				
(Weight Watchers)	9 oz	310	12	35
Cheese Manicotti				
(Weight Watchers)	9 oz	300	13	39
***Chicken Cacciatore Light**				
(Le Menu)	10 oz	260	8	28
***Chicken Fettucini**				
(Weight Watchers)	9 oz	300	10	30
Fettucine Alfredo:				
(Buitoni)	10 oz	440	26	53
(Stouffer's)	5 oz	270	18	60
Fettucine Carbonara (Buitoni)	10 oz	440	28	57
Fettucine with Meat				
(Green Giant)	10 oz	430	16	33
Fettucine Primavera: *(Buitoni)	10 oz	440	7	14
(Green Giant)	1	230	8	31
Lasagna:				
*(Green Giant)	9-½ oz	290	6	19
And Meat Sauce				
(Weight Watchers)	11 oz	340	14	37
(Stouffer's)	10 oz	385	14	33
Lasagna, Cheese				
(Weight Watchers)	12 oz	370	14	34
Lasagna, Chicken (Green Giant)	12 oz	640	32	45
Lasagna, Deep Dish:				
*(Buitoni)	11 oz	390	10	23
Meat (Buitoni)	11 oz	400	14	32
Lasagne, Spinach:				
(Buitoni)	9-½ oz	480	29	54
*(Green Giant)	12 oz	540	14	23
***Lasagna, Veal** (Lean Cuisine)	10 oz	280	8	26
Lasagna, Vegetable (Le Menu)	11 oz	360	19	48
***Lasagna, Zucchini**				
(Lean Cuisine)	11 oz	260	7	24
***Linguine and Clam Sauce**				
(Lean Cuisine)	10 oz	260	7	24

FOOD	MEASURE OR QUANTITY	CALORIES	FAT GRAMS	% FAT
Macaroni and Beef (Stouffer's)	6 oz	190	8	38
Macaroni and Cheese:				
(Banquet)	8 oz	340	17	45
(Green Giant)	9 oz	290	10	31
(Stouffer's)	6 oz	260	12	42
Manicotti				
*(Buitoni)	6 oz	270	9	30
(Le Menu)	8-½ oz	300	12	36
*And Sauce (Buitoni)	13 oz	420	12	26
Pasta Primavera:				
(Bird's Eye)	4 oz	121	5	37
(Weight Watchers)	9 oz	290	13	40
*Pasta Rigati (Weight Watchers)	11 oz	290	8	25
*Pasta Shells and Sauce				
(Banquet)	10 oz	310	8	23
*Ravioli, Cheese (Buitoni)	12 oz	440	12	25
Ravioli and Meat (Buitoni)	12 oz	520	18	31
Rotini Cheddar Gourmet				
(Green Giant)	1	220	11	45
Seafood Linguini (Weight Watchers)	9 oz	220	8	33
*Shells and Broccoli (Buitoni)	5 oz	150	3	18
Shells and Chicken (Stouffer's)	9 oz	320	14	39
Shells and Sauce (Buitoni)	10 oz	350	12	31
*Shells and Spinach (Buitoni)	6 oz	160	4	22
Shells, Beef and Spinach (Stouffer's)	9 oz	290	11	34
*Tortellini Provencal Gourmet (Green Giant)	1	210	5	21
Spaghetti and Meat Sauce:				
*(Stouffer's)	14 oz	445	12	24
*(Weight Watchers)	11 oz	280	7	22
Veal Primavera (Lean Cuisine)	10 oz	250	9	32
*Ziti (Buitoni)	10 oz	360	5	12

■ PASTA DISHES, PACKAGED
MADE ACCORDING TO PACKAGE
Fat Range = 23% to 46%
Average Fat = 36%

FOOD	MEASURE OR QUANTITY	CALORIES	FAT GRAMS	% FAT
Egg Noodle and Cheese (Kraft)	¾ cup	340	17	45
Egg Noodle and Chicken (Kraft)	¾ cup	240	10	38
Macaroni and Cheese:				
*Deluxe (Kraft)	¾ cup	260	8	28
(Kraft)	¾ cup	290	13	40
(Lipton)	½ cup	210	10	43
Noodles and Sauce (Lipton)	½ cup	190	9	43
Shells and Cheese (Velveeta)	¾ cup	260	10	35
*Spaghetti Dinner (Kraft)	1 cup	310	8	23
Spaghetti and Meat (Kraft)	1 cup	360	14	35

FOOD	MEASURE OR QUANTITY	CALORIES	FAT GRAMS	% FAT
Spiral Macaroni (Kraft)	¾ cup	330	17	46
*Tangy Italian Spaghetti (Kraft)	1 cup	310	8	23

■ **PASTA, PLAIN**

THE PORTIONS ARE DRY; COOKED, THE YIELD IS 1 CUP
Fat Range = 0% to 12%
Average Fat = 5%

FOOD	MEASURE OR QUANTITY	CALORIES	FAT GRAMS	% FAT
*Acini De Pepe (San Giorgio)	2 oz	210	1	4
*Alphabets (San Giorgio)	2 oz	210	1	4
*Angel Hair (Store Brand)	2 oz	210	1	4
*Bows (Store Brand)	2 oz	210	1	4
Capellini: *(San Giorgio)	2 oz	210	1	4
*(Store Brand)	2 oz	210	1	4
*Ditalini (San Giorgio)	2 oz	210	1	4
Elbow Macaroni:				
*(Mueller's)	2 oz	210	1	4
*(Store Brand)	2 oz	210	1	4
*Fettuccine (Store Brand)	2 oz	210	1	4
*Fusilli (San Giorgio)	2 oz	210	1	4
Lasagna:				
*(Mueller's)	2 oz	210	1	4
*(San Giorgio)	2 oz	210	1	4
*(Store Brand)	2 oz	210	1	4
Linguini:				
*(San Giorgio)	2 oz	210	1	4
*(Store Brand)	2 oz	210	1	4
*Linguini, Spinach				
(Store Brand)	2 oz	210	1	4
Macaroni:				
*(Buitoni)	2 oz	210	1	4
*(Mueller's)	2 oz	210	1	4
*(Ronzoni)	2 oz	210	1	4
*(Store Brand)	2 oz	210	1	4
*Macaroni, Spinach (Ronzoni)	2 oz	205	0	0
*Manicotti (Store Brand)	2 oz	210	1	4
*Mostaccioli (San Giorgio)	2 oz	210	1	4
*Noodles, Egg (Buitoni)	2 oz	220	3	12
*Noodles, Spinach (Buitoni)	2 oz	210	1	4
*Orzo (San Giorgio)	2 oz	210	1	4
*Pasta Romana (Buitoni)	2 oz	210	1	4
*Pastina (San Giorgio)	2 oz	210	1	4
*Racing Wheels (San Giorgio)	2 oz	210	1	4
*Ribbon Pasta (Pritikin)	2 oz	220	2	8
Rigatoni:				
*(San Giorgio)	2 oz	210	1	4
*(Store Brand)	2 oz	210	1	4
*Rotini (San Giorgio)	2 oz	210	1	4

FOOD	MEASURE OR QUANTITY	CALORIES	FAT GRAMS	% FAT
Shells:				
*(San Giorgio)	2 oz	210	1	4
*(Store Brand)	2 oz	210	1	4
Spaghetti:				
*(Buitoni)	2 oz	210	1	4
*(Mueller)	2 oz	210	1	4
*(Pritikin)	2 oz	170	1	5
*(Ronzoni)	2 oz	210	1	4
*(San Giorgio)	2 oz	210	1	4
*(Store Brand)	2 oz	210	1	4
*Tubetinni (San Giorgio)	2 oz	210	1	4
*Twists, Tri Color (Mueller's)	2 oz	210	1	4
Vermicelli:				
*(San Giorgio)	2 oz	210	1	4
*(Store Brand)	2 oz	210	1	4
Ziti:				
*(San Giorgio)	2 oz	210	1	4
*(Store Brand)	2 oz	210	1	4

■ POTATOES, PLAIN
Fat Range = 0%
Average Fat = 0%

FOOD	MEASURE OR QUANTITY	CALORIES	FAT GRAMS	% FAT
Baked:				
*No Skin	1	150	0	0
*With Skin	1	210	0	0
*With Skin, in Microwave	1	210	0	0
Raw:				
*Peeled	1	160	0	0
*With Skin	1	220	0	0

■ POTATOES, PREPARED
Fat Range = 0% to 69% Fat
Average Fat = 33%

FOOD	MEASURE OR QUANTITY	CALORIES	FAT GRAMS	% FAT
Au Gratin (Homemade)	½ cup	160	9	51
Baked:				
*Bacon (Oh Boy)	6 oz	116	3	23
Bacon, Cheddar Cheese (Idaho Original)	11 oz	980	74	68
*Broccoli and Cheese (Weight Watchers)	1	280	7	22

FOOD	MEASURE OR QUANTITY	CALORIES	FAT GRAMS	% FAT
*Cheese (Green Giant)	5 oz	200	6	27
Sour Cream (Bird's Eye)	5 oz	230	10	39
Sour Cream and Chives (Oh Boy)	6 oz	129	5	35
*Butter Sauce (Green Giant)	½ cup	80	2	22
Fries, French:				
(Bird's Eye)	3 oz	110	4	33
(Heinz)	3 oz	160	6	34
(Homemade)	10 pieces	160	8	45
*Lites (Ore Ida)	3 oz	90	2	20
Fries, Cottage:				
(Bird's Eye)	3 oz	120	5	38
(Ore Ida)	3 oz	140	6	39
Fries, Country Style (Ore Ida)	3 oz	110	4	33
Fries, Crinkle Cut:				
(Bird's Eye)	3 oz	110	4	33
*Lite (Ore Ida)	3 oz	90	2	20
(Ore Ida)	3 oz	120	5	38
Fries, Crispers (Ore Ida)	3 oz	240	15	56
Fries, Crispy Crowns (Ore Ida)	3 oz	150	8	48
Fries, Golden Patties (Ore Ida)	2-½ oz	130	10	69
Fries, Homestyle (Ore Ida)	3 oz	110	4	33
Fries, Onion:				
(Ore Ida)	3 oz	170	10	53
Tater Tots (Ore Ida)	3 oz	160	8	45
Fries, Pixie Crinkles (Ore Ida)	3 oz	160	10	56
Fries, Planks (Ore Ida)	3 oz	110	5	41
Fries, Puffs (Bird's Eye)	2-½ oz	190	12	57
Fries, Shoestring:				
(Bird's Eye)	3 oz	140	6	39
Lites (Ore Ida)	3 oz	90	4	40
(Ore Ida)	3 oz	160	7	39
Fries, Thin (Ore Ida)	3 oz	130	6	42
*Fries, Steak (Bird's Eye)	3 oz	110	3	25
Fries, Tater Tots (Ore Ida)	3 oz	160	7	39
Fries, Tiny Taters (Bird's Eye)	3 oz	200	12	54
Fries, Wedges (Ore Ida)	3 oz	100	4	36
Hash Browns:				
*(Bird's Eye)	3 oz	70	0	0
(Homemade)	½ cup	170	11	58
Microwave (Ore Ida)	2 oz	180	8	40
*(Ore Ida)	3 oz	70	0	0
Southern Style (Heinz)	3 oz	110	7	57
Mashed:				
(French's)	½ cup	130	6	42
(Homemade)	½ cup	120	5	38
(Hungry Jack)	½ cup	140	7	45
Mix, Au Gratin:				
(Betty Crocker)	½ cup	150	6	36
*(Lipton)	½ cup	108	0	0
*Mix, Beef and Mushroom (Lipton)	½ cup	95	0	0
*Mix, Cheddar Bacon (Lipton)	½ cup	106	1	8
*Mix, Cheddar and Broccoli (Lipton)	½ cup	104	1	9

FOOD	MEASURE OR QUANTITY	CALORIES	FAT GRAMS	% FAT
Mix, Cheese Scalloped (French's)	½ cup	140	5	32
*****Mix, Chicken Flavored** (Lipton)	½ cup	90	0	0
*****Mix, Chicken 'n Herbs** (Betty				
Crocker)	½ cup	120	4	30
Mix, Creamed:				
Oven (Betty Crocker)	½ cup	170	8	42
Saucepan (Betty Crocker)	½ cup	180	8	40
*****Mix, Creamy Italian with**				
Parmesan Cheese				
(French's)	½ cup	130	4	28
*****Mix, Creamy Stroganoff**				
(French's)	½ cup	130	4	28
*****Mix, German Salad** (Lipton)	½ cup	99	0	0
Mix, Hash Browns with Onions				
(Green Giant)	½ cup	150	6	36
*****Mix, Italiano** (Lipton)	½ cup	107	2	17
Mix, Mashed:				
(French's)	½ cup	140	7	45
Spuds (French's)	½ cup	140	7	45
*****Mix, Nacho** (Lipton)	½ cup	103	1	9
*****Mix, O'Brien** (Ore Ida)	3 oz	80	0	0
Mix, Potato Buds (Betty				
Crocker)	½ cup	130	6	42
*****Mix, Potato Salad** (Lipton)	½ cup	94	0	0
Mix, Scalloped:				
(Betty Crocker)	½ cup	140	6	39
*(French's)	½ cup	160	5	28
*(Lipton)	½ cup	102	2	18
With Cheese (French's)	½ cup	160	6	34
Mix, Sour Cream and Chives:				
(French's)	½ cup	150	6	36
(Green Giant)	½ cup	160	7	39
*(Lipton)	½ cup	113	2	16
Mix, Tangy Au Gratin (French's)	½ cup	140	6	39
Mix, Julienne (Betty Crocker)	½ cup	130	6	42
*****O'Brien** (Homemade)	1 cup	160	3	17
Pancakes, 2 large:				
(Homemade)	6 oz	300	14	42
(Mother's)	3 oz	120	6	45
*****Salad, German** (Joan of Arc)	½ cup	120	1	8
Salad (Joan of Arc)	½ cup	160	9	51
Scalloped (Homemade)	½ cup	100	5	45
Sweet Peas, Bacon in Cream				
Sauce (Green Giant)	½ cup	110	4	33

■ R I C E
Fat Range = 0%
Average Fat = 0%

FOOD	MEASURE OR QUANTITY	CALORIES	FAT GRAMS	% FAT
*Rice, Brown	1 cup	230	1	0
*Rice, White:	1 cup	220	0	0
*Enriched	1 cup	180	0	0
*Instant	1 cup	180	0	0
*Regular	1 cup	230	1	0

■ RICE DISHES
Fat Range = 0% to 43% Fat
Average Fat = 17%

FOOD	MEASURE OR QUANTITY	CALORIES	FAT GRAMS	% FAT
*Asparagus and Hollandaise Sauce (Lipton)	½ cup	125	0	0
Beef:				
*(Lipton)	½ cup	160	4	22
*(Minute Rice)	½ cup	150	4	24
*(Rice-A-Roni)	⅙ pkg	130	1	7
Broccoli and Cheese Sauce (Green Giant)	½ cup	140	6	39
*Brown, Beef Stock (Green Giant)	1 cup	300	8	24
*Cajun (Lipton)	½ cup	121	0	0
Chicken:				
*(Hain)	½ cup	100	1	9
*(Lipton)	½ cup	150	4	24
*(Minute Rice)	½ cup	150	4	24
*(Rice-A-Roni)	⅙ pkg	130	1	7
*Chinese Fried (Bird's Eye)	4 oz	100	0	0
*Florentine and Sauce (Lipton)	½ cup	135	1	7
*Fried (Minute Rice)	½ cup	160	5	28
Herb and Butter:				
(Green Giant)	½ cup	150	6	36
*(Lipton)	½ cup	160	5	28
Italian:				
*(Bird's Eye)	4 oz	130	1	7
*(Hain)	½ cup	130	2	14
*Macaroni and Cheddar (Rice-A-Roni)	⅙ pkg	190	2	9
Medley:				
*(Green Giant)	½ cup	120	3	22
*(Lipton)	½ cup	150	3	18
*Mushroom (Lipton)	½ cup	140	3	19
Mushrooms and Herbs, Long Grain (Lipton)	½ cup	42	2	43
*Noodle Roni (Rice-A-Roni)	⅙ pkg	130	3	21
*Oriental and Sauce (Lipton)	½ cup	131	1	7

FOOD	MEASURE OR QUANTITY	CALORIES	FAT GRAMS	% FAT
*Oriental Style (Bird's Eye)	4 oz	130	1	7
*Peas (Lipton)	½ cup	150	3	18
*Peas and Mushrooms				
(Bird's Eye)	2 oz	110	0	0
*Pilaf (Green Giant)	½ cup	120	2	15
Spanish:				
*(Bird's Eye)	4 oz	120	1	8
*(Hain)	½ cup	90	2	20
*(Heinz)	7-¼ oz	150	5	30
*(Lipton)	½ cup	140	3	19
*(Rice-A-Roni)	1/6 pkg	110	1	8
*(Van Camp)	1 cup	150	3	18
*Teriyaki (Hain)	½ cup	130	4	28
White:				
*Long Grain (Minute Rice)	½ cup	148	4	24
*(Minute Rice)	½ cup	148	4	24
*Wild (Minute Rice)	½ cup	148	4	24
Wild, Long Grain:				
*(Minute Rice)	½ cup	150	4	24
*Oriental (Lipton)	½ cup	120	0	0
*White (Green Giant)	½ cup	110	1	8

31. VEGETABLES

■ VEGETABLES
Fat Range = 0% to 22% Fat
Average Fat = 1%

FOOD	MEASURE OR QUANTITY	CALORIES	FAT GRAMS	% FAT
*Alfalfa Sprouts	1 cup	10	0	0
*Amaranth	1 cup	7	0	0
*Arrowhead	1	26	0	0
Artichoke:				
*Hearts	½ cup	40	0	0
*Whole, Large	1	80	0	0
*Asparagus	4	14	0	0
Bak Choi				
(See Cabbage, Chinese)				
Bamboo Shoots:				
*Kidney	½ cup	27	0	0
*Mung	½ cup	16	0	0
*Pinto	½ cup	33	0	0

FOOD	MEASURE OR QUANTITY	CALORIES	FAT GRAMS	% FAT
*Beets	½ cup	26	0	0
*Blackeye Peas, Boiled	1 cup	200	1	4
Broccoli:				
*Spears	½ cup	25	0	0
*Whole	½ cup	23	0	0
*Brussel Sprouts	½ cup	30	0	0
Cabbage, Green:				
*Boiled	½ cup	10	0	0
*Raw	½ cup	8	0	0
Cabbage Red:				
*Boiled	½ cup	16	0	0
*Raw	½ cup	10	0	0
Cabbage, Savoy:				
*Boiled	½ cup	18	0	0
*Raw	½ cup	10	0	0
Cabbage, Chinese:				
*Boiled	½ cup	10	0	0
*Raw	½ cup	5	0	0
Carrots:				
*Boiled	½ cup	35	0	0
*Raw	1	31	0	0
Cauliflower, Pieces:				
*Boiled	½ cup	15	0	0
*Raw	½ cup	12	0	0
Celery:				
*Boiled	½ cup	11	0	0
*Raw	1 stalk	6	0	0
*Chickory Greens, Raw	½ cup	21	0	0
*Chickory Witloof	½ cup	7	0	0
*Collards, Boiled	1 cup	30	0	0
*Coriander, Raw	½ cup	2	0	0
*Corn on the Cob	1 medium	80	0	0
*Corn, White	½ cup	90	1	10
*Corn, Yellow	½ cup	90	1	10
*Cowpeas, Boiled	1 cup	200	1	4
*Cucumber	½ cup	7	0	0
Dandelion Greens:				
*Boiled	½ cup	17	0	0
*Raw	½ cup	14	0	0
Dock:				
*Boiled	½ cup	14	0	0
*Raw	½ cup	15	0	0
Eggplant:				
*Boiled	½ cup	14	0	0
*Raw	½ cup	12	0	0
*Endive, Raw	½ cup	4	0	0
*Fuki	4 oz	10	0	0
Garden Cress:				
*Boiled	½ cup	17	0	0
*Raw	½ cup	8	0	0
*Garlic	3 cloves	14	0	0
*Ginger Root, Raw	¼ cup	20	0	0
*Gourd, Boiled	½ cup	25	0	0
*Green Beans, Boiled	½ cup	20	0	0
*Hominy	1 cup	140	1	6

FOOD	MEASURE OR QUANTITY	CALORIES	FAT GRAMS	% FAT
*Jerusalem Artichoke, Raw	1 cup	25	0	0
*Jew's Ear	1 cup	25	0	0
*Jute, Boiled	½ cup	16	0	0
*Kale, Boiled	½ cup	21	0	0
*Kohlrabi, Boiled	½ cup	24	0	0
Leeks:				
*Boiled	½ cup	16	0	0
*Raw	½ cup	32	0	0
*Lettuce, Bibb	2 leaves	2	0	0
*Lettuce, Boston	2 leaves	2	0	0
*Lettuce, Butterhead	2 leaves	2	0	0
*Lettuce, Iceberg	2 leaves	5	0	0
*Lettuce, Iceberg	1 head	70	0	0
*Lettuce, Iceberg, Shredded	½ cup	6	0	0
*Lettuce, Romaine	2 leaves	2	0	0
*Lotus Root	10 slices	45	0	0
Mushroom:				
*Boiled	½ cup	21	0	0
*Raw	½ cup	10	0	0
*Mushroom, Shitake	4	40	0	0
*Mustard Spinach, Raw	½ cup	17	0	0
*Mustard Green, Boiled	½ cup	12	0	0
*Okra, Boiled	½ cup	25	0	0
Onions:				
*Boiled	½ cup	30	0	0
*Raw	½ cup	27	0	0
*Parsley, Raw	½ cup	10	0	0
*Parsnips, Boiled	½ cup	63	0	0
Peas, Green:				
*Boiled	½ cup	70	0	0
*Raw	½ cup	65	0	0
*Peas, Split, Boiled	½ cup	115	0	0
*Peapod	1 cup	25	0	0
*Peppers, Hot Chili, Raw	1	18	0	0
*Peppers, Jalapeño	½ cup	12	0	0
Peppers, Sweet:				
*Boiled	½ cup	12	0	0
*Raw	½ cup	12	0	0
*Pigeon Peas, Boiled	1 cup	200	1	4
*Pimientos	1 oz	10	0	0
*Poi	½ cup	135	0	0
*Pokeberry Shoots	½ cup	16	0	0
*Potato, No Skin, Baked (See also, Potatoes)	1	150	0	0
*Potato, with Skin, Baked (See also, Potatoes)	1	210	0	0
*Potato, Peeled, Raw (See also, Potatoes)	1	90	0	0
*Potato, with Skin, Raw (See also, Potatoes)	1	220	0	0
*Pumpkin, Mashed, Boiled	½ cup	25	0	0
*Purslane, Boiled	½ cup	10	0	0
Radish:				
*Boiled	½ cup	13	0	0
*Raw	½ cup	7	0	0

FOOD	MEASURE OR QUANTITY	CALORIES	FAT GRAMS	% FAT
*Rhubarb, Raw	½ cup	30	0	0
*Rice, Brown,				
Cooked (See also, Rice)	1 cup	230	1	4
*Rice, White,				
Cooked (See also, Rice)	1 cup	220	0	0
*Rutabaga, Boiled	½ cup	30	0	0
*Sauerkraut, Raw	2 oz	12	0	0
*Seaweed, Agar, Raw	3-½ oz	26	0	0
*Seaweed, Irishmoss, Raw	3-½ oz	50	0	0
*Seaweed, Kelp, Raw	3-½ oz	44	0	0
*Seaweed, Laver, Raw	3-½ oz	35	0	0
*Seaweed, Tangle, Raw	3-½ oz	44	0	0
*Seaweed, Wakame, Raw	3-½ oz	45	0	0
*Shallots, Raw	1 T	7	0	0
*Snap Beans, Boiled	½ cup	20	0	0
Spinach, New Zealand:				
*Boiled	½ cup	11	0	0
*Raw	½ cup	4	0	0
*Squash, Acorn, Baked	½ cup	60	0	0
*Squash, Butternut, Boiled	½ cup	40	0	0
*Squash, Crookneck, Boiled	½ cup	18	0	0
*Squash, Hubbard, Boiled	½ cup	50	1	18
*Squash, Scallop, Boiled	½ cup	14	0	0
*Squash, Spaghetti, Boiled	½ cup	25	0	0
Squash, Summer, All Types:				
*Boiled	½ cup	18	0	0
*Raw	½ cup	14	0	0
*Squash, Winter, Baked	½ cup	40	1	22
*Squash, Zucchini, Boiled	½ cup	14	0	0
*Succotash, Boiled	½ cup	110	1	8
*Swamp Cabbage, Boiled	½ cup	10	0	0
Sweet Potato:				
*Baked	1	120	0	0
*Mashed, Boiled	½ cup	170	1	5
*Taro, Cooked	½ cup	95	0	0
*Tomato, Green	1	30	0	0
*Tomato Paste	½ cup	110	1	8
*Tomato Paste	6 oz	150	0	0
*Tomato Puree	1 cup	100	0	0
*Tomato, Stewed	½ cup	35	0	0
*Tomato, Red	1	24	0	0
*Tomato Wedges	½ cup	30	0	0
*Turnip, Boiled	½ cup	14	0	0
Turnip Greens:				
*Boiled	½ cup	15	0	0
*Raw	½ cup	7	0	0
*Water Chestnut, Chinese, Raw	½ cup	70	0	0
*Watercress, Raw	½ cup	2	0	0
*Waxgourd, Boiled	½ cup	11	0	0
*Yam, Boiled	½ cup	80	0	0

■ VEGETABLE DISHES

Fat Range = 0% to 69% Fat
Average Fat = 29%

FOOD	MEASURE OR QUANTITY	CALORIES	FAT GRAMS	% FAT
Asparagus in Butter Sauce				
(Green Giant)	½ cup	70	4	51
Broccoli with Almonds				
(Bird's Eye)	3-1/3 oz	50	3	54
*Broccoli and Carrots				
(Bird's Eye)	3 oz	30	0	0
Broccoli, Carrots and Pasta				
(Bird's Eye)	3 oz	90	4	40
*Broccoli and Cauliflower				
(Green Giant)	½ cup	60	1	15
*Broccoli, Cauliflower & Carrots in Cheese Sauce				
(Green Giant)	½ cup	60	2	30
*Broccoli, Cauliflower and Red Peppers				
(Bird's Eye)	3 oz	25	0	0
Broccoli and Cheese Sauce:				
(Bird's Eye)	5 oz	120	7	52
*(Green Giant)	½ cup	70	2	26
(Stouffer's)	4-½ oz	130	8	55
*Broccoli, Corn and Red Peppers (Bird's Eye)	3 oz	60	2	30
*Broccoli, Green Beans, Onions and Red Peppers				
(Bird's Eye)	3 oz	25	0	0
*Broccoli Spears in Butter Sauce (Green Giant)	½ cup	40	1	22
*Broccoli and Water Chestnuts				
(Bird's Eye)	3 oz	30	0	0
*Brussel Sprouts in Butter Sauce (Green Giant)	½ cup	60	1	15
*Brussel Sprouts, Cauliflower and Carrots (Bird's Eye)	3 oz	30	0	0
Brussel Sprouts in Cheese Sauce:				
(Bird's Eye)	4-½ oz	120	6	45
*(Green Giant)	½ cup	80	2	22
*Carrots in Butter Sauce				
(Green Giant)	½ cup	80	1	11
*Carrots, Sweet Peas, Onions				
(Bird's Eye)	3 oz	50	0	0
Cauliflower and Almonds				
(Bird's Eye)	3 oz	40	2	45
*Cauliflower and Carrots				
(Green Giant)	½ cup	60	0	0
Cauliflower in Cheese Sauce:				
(Bird's Eye)	½ cup	114	6	47
(Bird's Eye)	5 oz	120	7	52
Cheddar (Green Giant)	½ cup	70	3	39
*(Green Giant)	½ cup	60	2	30
(Pillsbury)	½ cup	70	4	51

FOOD	MEASURE OR QUANTITY	CALORIES	FAT GRAMS	% FAT
*Cauliflower and Green Beans				
(Green Giant)	½ cup	16	0	0
*Cauliflower, Green Beans and Corn				
(Bird's Eye)	3 oz	35	0	0
Coleslaw (Homemade)	½ cup	45	2	40
*Corn in Butter Sauce				
(Green Giant)	½ cup	100	2	18
Corn, Cream Style:				
*(Green Giant)	½ cup	100	1	9
*(Del Monte)	½ cup	80	1	11
*(Homemade)	½ cup	100	1	9
Corn in Cream Sauce				
(Green Giant)	½ cup	130	5	35
Corn and Green Beans with Pasta				
(Bird's Eye)	3 oz	110	5	41
Corn on the Cob:				
*(Bird's Eye)	1	120	1	8
*(Green Giant)	1	140	1	6
Corn Pudding (Homemade)	1 cup	300	14	42
*Corn, Sweet (Bird's Eye)	3 oz	80	1	11
*Corn, White in Butter Sauce				
(Green Giant)	½ cup	100	2	18
*Green Beans, Carrots and				
Onions (Bird's Eye)	½ cup	45	0	0
*Green Beans, Cauliflower and				
Carrots (Bird's Eye)	½ cup	25	0	0
Green Beans in Mushroom				
Cream Sauce (Bird's Eye)	½ cup	80	4	45
Green Beans with Toasted				
Almonds (Green Giant)	3 oz	50	2	36
Hummus (Homemade)	1 cup	450	22	44
*Lima Beans in Butter Sauce				
(Green Giant)	½ cup	120	2	15
Mixed:				
*(Bird's Eye)	3 oz	60	0	0
*(Green Giant)	½ cup	60	0	0
*(Libby's)	½ cup	40	0	0
*(S&W)	½ cup	35	0	0
Mixed, Bavarian Style				
(Bird's Eye)	3 oz	110	6	49
Mixed, Chinese Style:				
(Bird's Eye)	3 oz	80	5	56
(Green Giant)	½ cup	60	3	45
Mixed, Far Eastern Style				
(Bird's Eye)	3 oz	80	5	56
Mixed, Italian Style (Bird's Eye)	3 oz	110	7	57
Mixed, Japanese Style				
(Bird's Eye)	3 oz	100	6	54
Mixed, Mexican Style				
(Bird's Eye)	3 oz	120	6	45
Mixed, New England Style				
(Bird's Eye)	3 oz	130	7	48
Mixed, Onion Sauce (Bird's Eye)	2-½ oz	100	5	45
Mixed, San Francisco Style				
(Bird's Eye)	3 oz	100	5	45

FOOD	MEASURE OR QUANTITY	CALORIES	FAT GRAMS	% FAT
Mixed, Stir Fry:				
*Chinese Style (Bird's Eye)	3 oz	30	0	0
*Japanese Style (Bird's Eye)	3 oz	30	0	0
Mushrooms in Butter Sauce:				
*Canned (Green Giant)	2 oz	30	1	30
Frozen (Green Giant)	½ cup	70	4	51
Mushrooms in Creamy Sauce				
(Green Giant)	1	220	11	45
Onions in Cheese Sauce				
(Green Giant)	½ cup	90	5	50
Onions in Cream Sauce				
(Bird's Eye)	3 oz	110	6	49
***Peas in Butter Sauce**				
(Green Giant)	½ cup	90	1	10
Peas and Carrots:				
*(Del Monte)	½ cup	50	0	0
*(Libby's)	½ cup	50	0	0
*(S&W)	½ cup	50	0	0
Peas, Carrots and Onions:				
*(Bird's Eye)	3 oz	70	0	0
*(Le Sueur)	½ cup	90	3	30
***Peas and Cauliflower**				
(Green Giant)	½ cup	40	0	0
Peas in Cream Sauce:				
(Bird's Eye)	3 oz	130	7	48
(Green Giant)	½ cup	100	4	36
***Peas and Onions** (S&W)	½ cup	60	1	15
Peas and Onions in Cheese				
Sauce (Bird's Eye)	5 oz	140	5	32
***Peas, Pea Pods and Water**				
Chestnuts in Butter	½ cup	80	2	22
Peas, Potatoes in Cream Sauce				
(Bird's Eye)	2-½ oz	140	7	45
Potatoes (See Potatoes)				
Salad, Creamy Pasta				
(Bird's Eye)	½ cup	140	6	39
Salad, Creamy Ranch				
(Bird's Eye)	½ cup	170	9	48
***Salad, German Potato**				
(Bird's Eye)	½ cup	110	3	25
Salad, Italian (Bird's Eye)	½ cup	190	11	52
Salad, Three Bean				
(Bird's Eye)	½ cup	160	11	62
***Sauerkraut, Canned**				
(Del Monte)	½ cup	25	0	0
Spinach, Butter Sauce				
(Green Giant)	½ cup	50	2	36
Spinach, Creamed:				
(Bird's Eye)	3 oz	60	3	45
(Green Giant)	½ cup	70	3	39
***Spinach and Water Chestnuts**				
(Bird's Eye)	3 oz	25	0	0
***Stew Vegetables** (Ore Ida)	3 oz	60	0	0
Succotash:				
*(Libby's)	½ cup	80	1	11
*(S&W)	½ cup	80	1	11

FOOD	MEASURE OR QUANTITY	CALORIES	FAT GRAMS	% FAT
Tomato Paste, Italian Style:				
*Contadina	2 oz	70	1	13
*Hunt's	2 oz	50	0	0
*With Mushrooms (Contadina)	2 oz	60	1	15
*Tomato, Red Kosher (Claussen)	1 oz	5	0	0
*Zucchini in Tomato Sauce				
(Del Monte)	½ cup	30	0	0

DR. LOWELL'S LABEL FAT PERCENTAGE FINDER

CALORIES

	50	75	100	125	150	175	200	225	250	275	300	325	350	375	400
F 1	18	12	9	7	6	5	4	4	4	3	3	3	3	2	2
2	36	24	18	14	12	10	9	8	7	7	6	6	5	5	4
A 3	54	36	27	22	18	15	14	12	11	10	9	8	8	7	7
T 4	72	48	36	29	24	21	18	16	14	13	12	11	10	10	9
5	90	60	45	36	30	26	22	20	18	16	15	14	13	12	11
G 6	100	72	54	43	36	31	27	24	22	20	18	17	15	14	14
R 7		84	63	50	42	36	32	28	25	23	21	19	18	17	16
A 8		96	72	58	48	41	36	32	29	26	24	22	21	19	18
M 9			81	65	54	46	40	36	32	29	27	25	23	22	20
S 10			90	72	60	51	45	40	36	33	30	28	26	24	22
11			99	79	66	57	50	44	40	36	33	30	28	26	25
12				86	72	62	54	48	43	39	36	33	31	29	27
13				94	78	67	58	52	47	43	39	36	33	31	29
14					84	72	63	56	50	46	42	39	36	34	32
15					90	77	68	60	54	49	45	42	39	36	34
F 16					96	82	72	64	58	52	48	44	41	38	36
A 17						87	76	68	61	56	51	47	44	41	38
T 18						93	81	72	65	59	54	50	46	43	40
19						98	86	76	68	62	57	53	49	46	43
20							90	80	72	65	60	55	51	48	45
G 21							94	84	76	69	63	58	54	50	47
R 22							99	88	79	72	66	61	57	53	50
A 23								92	83	75	69	64	59	55	52
M 24								96	86	79	72	66	62	58	54
S 25								100	90	82	75	69	64	60	56
26									94	85	78	72	67	62	58
27									97	88	81	75	69	65	61
28									100	92	84	78	72	67	63
29										95	87	80	75	70	65
30										98	90	83	77	72	68

(Right side vertical label: PERCENT FAT)

USING THE FAT FINDER

1. Calories from nutritional panel are found on top line
2. Fat Grams from nutritional panel are found along the side
3. Join a straight line from calories to fat grams to find percent fat
4. *PICK FOODS THAT ARE 30% FAT OR LESS*
5. Take this copy when shopping
6. EXAMPLE: 150 CALORIES WITH 5 GRAMS FAT = 30% FAT

ABOUT THE AUTHOR

Bruce K. Lowell, M.D., is an internist and founder of the Lowell Metabolic Program, a system specializing in weight and health-risk management, with offices in Manhattan and Queens. He has been a guest on national television and radio shows, and he lectures to groups around the country.